Human Rights in Psychiatry

Dirk Richter

Human Rights in Psychiatry

Prospects and Dilemmas of Abolishing Coercion in Mental Health Care

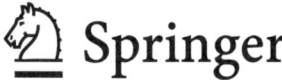 Springer

Dirk Richter
Department of Health Professions
Bern University of Applied Sciences
Bern, Switzerland

ISBN 978-3-031-98634-5   ISBN 978-3-031-98635-2 (eBook)
https://doi.org/10.1007/978-3-031-98635-2

© The Editor(s) (if applicable) and The Author(s), under exclusive license to Springer Nature Switzerland AG 2025

This work is subject to copyright. All rights are solely and exclusively licensed by the Publisher, whether the whole or part of the material is concerned, specifically the rights of translation, reprinting, reuse of illustrations, recitation, broadcasting, reproduction on microfilms or in any other physical way, and transmission or information storage and retrieval, electronic adaptation, computer software, or by similar or dissimilar methodology now known or hereafter developed.
The use of general descriptive names, registered names, trademarks, service marks, etc. in this publication does not imply, even in the absence of a specific statement, that such names are exempt from the relevant protective laws and regulations and therefore free for general use.
The publisher, the authors and the editors are safe to assume that the advice and information in this book are believed to be true and accurate at the date of publication. Neither the publisher nor the authors or the editors give a warranty, expressed or implied, with respect to the material contained herein or for any errors or omissions that may have been made. The publisher remains neutral with regard to jurisdictional claims in published maps and institutional affiliations.

This Springer imprint is published by the registered company Springer Nature Switzerland AG
The registered company address is: Gewerbestrasse 11, 6330 Cham, Switzerland

If disposing of this product, please recycle the paper.

Acknowledgements

This book is the result of numerous discussions and controversies with many participants. I was able to present various versions of my thoughts at conferences and meetings of the "European Violence in Psychiatry Research Group" and the COST network "Fostering and Strengthening Approaches to Reducing Coercion in European Mental Health Services". I would like to thank EVIPRG and FOSTREN colleagues for their constructive criticism.

Without the experiences and discussions at the Division of Nursing at Bern University of Applied Sciences and at the Centre for Psychiatric Rehabilitation at the University Psychiatric Services Bern, this book would probably never have been written. I would particularly like to thank Sabine Hahn, Christian Burr, Daniel Schärer and Walter Gekle.

Sabine Rühle Andersson, a service user and research associate in my research group at Bern University of Applied Sciences, and Anastasia Theodoridou, psychiatrist and psychotherapist at Psychiatrie Baselland, Liestal, read the entire German manuscript and saved me from many errors, inadequacies and inaccuracies. Thank you very much for your support.

The same thanks also go to my son (and psychologist) Tim and to my wife Doris, who also took the effort to proofread the entire German manuscript. Doris has been not only a wonderful life partner for more than 40 years but also a sparring partner in matters of coercion and psychiatry. From her many years of experience as a social worker, she has repeatedly pointed out counterexamples as well as practical problems and dilemmas in my argumentation and thus made a decisive contribution to sharpening my thoughts and to the clarity of the text.

This book has been published previously in a slightly modified version in a German-language open access edition by Psychiatrie-Verlag, Cologne, Germany. Karin Koch from Psychiatrie-Verlag carefully edited the German-language manuscript and streamlined the arguments. I would also like to thank her for this.

The—hopefully not too many—remaining errors and ambiguities are solely attributable to me.

Contents

1 Human Rights and Coercion in Mental Health Care: Concepts, Data and Terminology.............................. 1
  1.1 Introduction 1
  1.2 Psychiatric Coercion: What Exactly Is it?..................... 3
  1.3 The Extent of Coercion Against People with Psychosocial Problems in the Present Day 5
  1.4 Towards a Nondiscriminatory and Non-pejorative Terminology.... 8
  1.5 The Plan of the Book.. 11
  References.. 11

2 Human Rights and Psychiatric Coercion: The Legitimisation Problem for (Social) Psychiatry............................. 15
  2.1 Introduction 15
  2.2 Human Rights and the Social Model of Disability 18
  2.3 The Controversy Surrounding the Use of Coercion in Social Psychiatry 21
  2.4 The Controversy Surrounding Medical Aid in Dying for People with Psychosocial Problems........................ 23
  2.5 Conclusion: The Decision-Making Dilemma of (Social) Psychiatry.. 26
  References.. 27

3 The Legitimisation of Psychiatric Measures Against a Person's Will... 31
  3.1 Introduction 31
  3.2 Coercion in Psychiatric Care: The Institution-Centred Phase 31
  3.3 From the Institution-Centred Phase to the Person-Centred Phase 35
  3.4 The Legitimisation of Coercion in the Person-Centred Phase 38
  3.5 Conclusion: The Legitimisation of Coercion in Psychiatry: The Clinical-Ethical-Legal Stalemate............. 41
  References.. 42

4	**Psychiatric Coercion: Ethical Conditions and Empirical Data**	45
	4.1 Introduction	45
	4.2 Condition 1: Is Coercion for the Benefit of the Person Concerned?	46
	4.3 Condition 2: Is the Least Possible Restriction Used, and Is It Used as a Last Resort?	50
	4.4 Condition 3: Is Psychiatric Treatment Effective?	52
	4.5 Condition 4: Can the Autonomy of the Persons Concerned Be Restored?	55
	4.6 Conclusion: Ethical Assumptions and Empirical Data	57
	References	57
5	**Mental Disorder: What Is It and How Valid Is the Definition?**	63
	5.1 Introduction	63
	5.2 Is There Even a Human Psyche?	64
	5.3 Social Change and Individualisation	67
	5.4 Individualisation and Psychologisation	69
	5.5 Interaction of Sensitivities and Diagnostic Classifications	70
	5.6 Mentally "Ill" or "Not Ill": Historical Developments Between Eugenics and Psychiatry	72
	5.7 The Problem of Demarcation	74
	5.8 The Problem of Psychological Dysfunction	77
	5.9 Can a Distinction Be Made Between Different Mental Disorders?	79
	5.10 Conclusion: Human Rights and the Real Construct of Mental Disorder	81
	References	83
6	**Psychosocial Problems: The Spectrum Model**	87
	6.1 Introduction	87
	6.2 From Neurodiversity to Neurocognitive Diversity	88
	6.3 From Neurocognitive Diversity to Sociodiversity	91
	6.4 Psychosocial Problems in a Socio-diverse Context	94
	6.5 Psychosocial Problems: The Spectrum Model	95
	6.6 From a Psychological Phenomenon to a Psychosocial Problem	97
	6.7 Mentally Ill or Not: The Assessment Spectrum	99
	6.8 Conclusion: Disease Definition as a Perspective Construct	102
	References	102
7	**Human Rights-Based Psychosocial Support**	107
	7.1 Introduction	107
	7.2 Human Rights Development in Mental Health Care	107
	7.3 What Support Preferences Do People with Psychosocial Problems Have?	108
	7.4 From Shared Decision-Making to Supported Decision-Making	110

	7.5	Supported Decision-Making: Preference over Evidence	111
	7.6	Human Rights-Based Psychosocial Support: Person-Centred and Preference-Based.	113
	7.7	Conclusions: Building Blocks of Person-Centred Support	122
	References	122

8 Psychosocial Support Without Coercion: Consequences, Dilemmas and Possible Ways Out 127
    8.1 Introduction 127
    8.2 Consequences of a Preference-Oriented Self-Declaration of Ill/Not Ill. 128
    8.3 Consequences of Preference-Based Psychosocial Support 130
    8.4 Harm to Others in a Psychosocial Support Programme Without Coercion 131
    8.5 Self-Harm in a Psychosocial Support Programme Without Coercion. 132
    8.6 Dementia and Psychosocial Support Without Coercion 134
    8.7 Conclusions: Towards Psychosocial Support Without Coercion. 135
    References. 135

9 Epilogue: On the Way to a Post-liberal Psychiatry? 139
    9.1 Text. 139
    References. 140

Human Rights and Coercion in Mental Health Care: Concepts, Data and Terminology

1.1 Introduction

In the following chapters, I will try to explain why coercion can no longer be justified in mental health care, including mental health nursing, and what a psychiatry without coercion could look like. I hate to admit it, but during my practical time in mental health nursing in the 1980s, I too worked on closed wards and took part in involuntary admissions as well as in more extensive physical coercive measures such as mechanical restraint and forced medication. Being involved in these measures was the most unpleasant part of the job—I hated it. It was not primarily the risk of being physically harmed during a coercive measure that made it unpleasant. Rather, it was against my personal and professional convictions.

From today's perspective, it is time to take a critical look at my own involvement in coercive measures. It is also time, and this is not just my personal opinion [1], to apologise for my own involvement to the people who had to suffer under the measures taken against their will. Of course, back in the days, I would have had virtually no opportunity to work against the system of coercive measures. In the mental health nursing profession, you were—and still are—part of a professional hierarchy and part of a chain of medical orders.

Additionally, I was able to justify it to myself, as I was dealing with people with mental illnesses who were in danger to themselves or others. Moreover, the measures were ultimately for the benefit of the patients, or so I thought. At the time, hardly anyone doubted this practice. It was a necessary evil if you worked in psychiatric hospitals. Moreover, as was also noted at the time, there was virtually no empirical research on these problems until well into the 1990s [2], on the basis of which the practice of psychiatric coercion could have been questioned.

A few publications, for example, by the psychiatrist and psychoanalyst Thomas Szasz, were of a more fundamental nature and, in addition to the existence of mental illness, doubted state intervention from a right-wing libertarian position [3, 4]. Szasz was one of the most prominent, influential and controversial researchers who considered the use of coercion in psychiatry to be illegitimate. His reasoning was quite simple: "Mental illnesses" are not real illnesses, as they do not—like physical illnesses—exhibit organic damage. This also removed the legitimisation of coercive measures against people diagnosed as "mentally ill".

As the German philosopher Thomas Schramme [5] noted, Szasz certainly asked the right questions—and many of the questions he posed (Can coercion be legitimised? What is actually a "mental illness"?) will crop up again in this book. However, Szasz was also a man of his scientific times, and, as of today, many of his theories would be regarded as empirically unfounded. This includes, for example, the strict separation of physical and mental phenomena, which is now considered disproved. Mental phenomena are inconceivable without physical processes; today, we have more of a problem as to whether we can still speak of a human psyche at all—but more so in the course of the book.

In the meantime, empirical research in the neurosciences and psychology has investigated many issues that are relevant to the question of the legitimisation of coercion and has produced results that allow the question of legitimisation to be answered differently today; hence, the emphasis on the fact that coercive measures are *no longer* justifiable. There are numerous studies and other results of basic research in psychiatry, against the background of which at least considerable doubts arise about the use of coercion in psychiatry. I discuss these results in detail in Chaps. 4 and 5. In my view, however, the research results go beyond the doubts. They delegitimise psychiatric measures against the will of the persons concerned. To name just two central facts, we cannot validly define mental illness and differentiate it from healthy conditions, and it is clear that the measures are predominantly not for the benefit of the people affected by them. Essentially, my aim is to show that psychiatry cannot fulfil the ethical and medical criteria it has set itself for the justification of coercion. To emphasise this clearly, the same criteria that I am criticising here as inadequate for the use of psychiatric coercion are of course also lacking in the practice of mental health nursing. Nursing professionals must also face the criticism that they do not sufficiently observe ethical standards. They must consider what consequences this should have for their own actions.

Psychiatric coercion is not just a matter of the recent past but also a connection that has been known for centuries. The involuntary segregation of people with certain behaviours that were not tolerated by other people has been handed down in Europe since the Middle Ages. As the sociologist and historian Andrew Scull reports in his cultural history of "madness", there were individual institutions that detained such people from as early as the thirteenth or fourteenth centuries [6]. However, the massive expansion of such institutions did not take place until many centuries later, as will be described in more detail in Chap. 3.

Coercion in psychiatric care is still a fundamental problem. As shown in the course of this chapter, there is evidence from various countries that involuntary placements in psychiatric institutions have increased in recent years. However, the use of coercion in psychiatric care has been subject to massive and increasing criticism, particularly in the last 20 years. The background of this is the United Nations Convention on the Rights of Persons with Disabilities of 2006 (hereinafter UN

CRPD) [7]. The Convention views the use of measures against the will of people with physical and mental disabilities from a human rights perspective and generally categorises these measures as violations of human rights. Although individual passages of the Convention, which has been ratified by almost all countries in the world, are not entirely clear and are also the subject of controversial debate in some areas [8], the objective is clear: ultimately, it is about abolishing coercion in the care of people with disabilities, which in the Convention also includes people who are considered to be mentally disordered or ill from a medical perspective.

The publication of the UN CRPD and various other documents from the human rights movement in the United Nations triggered a massive debate about whether and how measures against people's will can be justified psychiatrically. There has been considerable resistance to the Convention and its overall thrust, particularly from international medical professional organisations. This resistance intensified when the United Nations Special Rapporteur categorised coercive psychiatric measures as torture [9]. Both clinical and, interestingly, human rights arguments were put forward against the goal of abolishing coercion. From a clinical perspective, "mental disorders" are associated with a risk of impaired judgement, which could justify measures against the person's will. In terms of human rights, those in favour of psychiatric coercion argued that it could also protect, for example, the right to health or the right to life [10].

1.2 Psychiatric Coercion: What Exactly Is it?

Basically, psychiatric coercion is quite easy to define: it is any measure taken against a person's will that is necessarily justified by the existence of a diagnosed mental disorder, a mental "weakness" or an intellectual disability. As is well-known, a distinction is usually made between necessary and sufficient conditions. Such a distinction is important, in particular, regarding formal legal justifications. Sufficient legitimisation generally also requires potential danger or risk to oneself or others that has already occurred or is highly likely to occur. The justifications vary considerably from country to country.

When I wrote at the beginning of the previous paragraph that the definition is basically simple, this implies that on closer inspection, it is actually quite difficult. There is still no generally recognised taxonomy of psychiatric coercion, i.e. a classification scheme that helps distinguish between different aspects of compulsion.

In the context of psychiatric coercion, formal and informal measures are usually assumed [11]. *Formal coercion* implies a legal decision on the basis of a medical assessment. Depending on the jurisdiction and the facts of the case, there may be a court hearing and a legal decision, but often, a doctor's order is already legally binding. On the basis of these decisions, a person can be admitted to a hospital against their will, and under certain circumstances, they can also be subjected to further coercive measures, such as restraint with belts, seclusion/isolation in a separate room or an injection against their will. The legal requirements for this vary from country to country and are sometimes also inconsistent within a country, for example, in federal structures in the United States, Germany or Switzerland. Placement in a forensic facility must also be categorised as formal coercion.

Informal coercion, also known as "soft coercion" [12], does not, as the name suggests, involve formal medical or legal measures. Here, communicative pressure is usually exerted on a person by professionals or legal representatives to achieve a certain behaviour [13]. Many formally voluntary stays in hospitals are based on such informal coercion. This ranges from a reference to enforcing a corresponding order in court if admission to the hospital is not voluntary to threats of physical violence, which—even if formally inadmissible—occur in psychiatric institutions [14]. The reference to possible formal coercion and the fact that psychiatric staff do in fact have such powers interweaves formal and informal coercion; and this is one of the issues that is difficult to distinguish.

In addition, there is another form of coercion in the mental health care system that has hardly been recognised as such and—as far as I have researched—has never been described in this way. This is *social or administrative coercion*, which the area of psychiatric rehabilitation, for example, is confronted with on an almost daily basis. Social coercion is used when certain decisions are made for people from an administrative perspective that forces them into certain life situations. This happens, for example, when legal representatives or insurance companies prevent people from utilising certain support services. One of the consequences of this is that the people affected have to work in workshops for people with disabilities instead of trying to gain a foothold in the primary labour market. Similarly, instead of living independently in their own home, they may have to live in a sheltered housing community.

The latter facts correspond to the distinction between negative and positive freedom introduced by the philosopher Isaiah Berlin [15]. "Negative freedom" refers to the absence of influence on one's personal life. "Positive freedom" refers to the possibility of developing and unfolding one's own life. While negative freedom can be associated with the absence of formal coercion, positive freedom is lost when administrative decisions restrict development opportunities.

The forms of coercion just described can be found in all countries of the world. A special form of psychiatric coercion can also be found in many low- and middle-income countries (LMICs). This refers to the segregation of people ordered or carried out by families or village elders, who are kept in cages or chained [16, 17]. These practices, which are based on long traditions, are particularly common in rural areas where psychiatric care is not available and where there is a pronounced stigmatisation of "unusual" behaviour. These practices are reminiscent of the practices known from European antiquity, in which the family had the task of keeping people with conspicuous behaviour away from the community [18].

Table 1.1 summarises the circumstances of the various types of coercion.

Another factor in this context is the subjective experience of coercion. Whether and to what extent the behaviour of employees is experienced as coercion depends not least on the context of the experience. Informal coercion can also be experienced if no measure is threatened, but the person concerned can expect this to be the case [19]. I have already questioned elsewhere [20] whether the distinction between

Table 1.1 Forms of coercion in psychiatric care

Forced type	Medium	Result	Examples
Formal	Medical-legal decision	Loss of freedom and autonomy	Forced hospitalisation, restraint, seclusion/isolation, compulsory treatment, placement in a forensic facility
Informal	Threatening and pressurising communication	Loss of autonomy	Formal voluntary but enforced intake of medication with the indication that otherwise a formal coercive measure could be taken
Social/administrative	Medical-administrative decision	Deprivation of social development possibilities and opportunities	Decision by an authority or a legal representative in favour of a specific housing situation against the will of the person concerned
Traditional/family	Decision of the family or a community	Isolation from social contacts	Restraining affected persons using chains or cages

positive and negative freedom is sufficient for a taxonomy, as proposed in the literature [21]. The last word has not yet been spoken about a taxonomy of coercion.

1.3 The Extent of Coercion Against People with Psychosocial Problems in the Present Day

How common is coercion in psychiatric care? Formal psychiatric coercion is assumed to affect several million people worldwide every year. A recent analysis of published data on coercive measures from countries in the Western world has shown that a median of 120 out of 100,000 people are affected by formal measures each year [22]. Extrapolated to the population of the 27 EU member states, this would already affect more than half a million people per year in this relatively small part of the world. However, there is a lack of relevant data and up-to-date statistics in many countries, which, in my view, is a scandal.

A comparative study of the incidence of involuntary hospitalisations in Europe, Australia and New Zealand revealed that these admissions increased significantly in most countries between 2008 and 2017 [23]. As an update, I undertook my own nonsystematic literature search of time series on involuntary measures in mental health care after this period. This revealed the following picture. Increases in involuntary measures have been reported in Brazil [24], Italy [25], Croatia [26], Switzerland [27], Canada [28–30], Australia [31], England and Wales [32–34], Scotland [35], Germany [36, 37] and the Netherlands [38]. Different developments have been reported in the United States. The majority of states reported an increase in coercive measures, whereas a minority of states reported a decrease [39].

Relatively unchanged figures were reported from China [40] and Finland [41]. In New Zealand, there was no significant change across the board, but there were differences in various forms of restraint, namely, a decrease in seclusion/isolation but an increase in community treatment orders [42]. Significant decreases in coercive measures were reported in Ireland [43] and Oregon, USA [44].

This means that there has been an overall increase in psychiatric coercion in many countries in recent decades, at least according to published data. However, these data are fraught with considerable methodological problems, particularly with regard to international comparability. The relevant factors here include different legal frameworks, different data collection procedures and problems with data quality [45]. In addition, these data are generally not transferable to low- and middle-income countries [22].

In my view, the expansion of formal coercion beyond the already extensive forms is worrying. I am not referring to the return of politically punitive psychiatry in Russia [46] on the basis of what is described as "archaic" care [47] or the abuse of psychiatry in Iran [48]. Rather, it refers to political intentions in the United States to consider homelessness alone as an indication of compulsory hospitalisation [49]. This also refers to the extension of coercion to the outpatient sector, where community treatment orders are increasingly seen as a "humane" alternative to placement in a psychiatric hospital [50].

This expansion can also be seen in another sector, namely, forensic hospitalisation. For several decades, the number of forensic psychiatric beds in the Western world has increased significantly [51], and this has also been the case in Germany, for example, until recently [52]. A general methodological difficulty with these data is the inconsistent collection from different sectors of care. For example, forensic hospitalisation is not usually included in health care systems research. A corresponding data analysis from various European countries has shown that a comparatively large number of people are forensically detained in the Netherlands and Belgium, whereas relatively few people are in Spain and Italy [53]. In addition to aspects of care systems, the extent to which different legal traditions prevail in different countries, particularly in the area of forensics, must also be considered [54].

Another area that goes hand in hand with psychiatric coercion in various respects is a distinct black box from a scientific perspective. This refers to the instrument of guardianship. Even special data collection by specialists in this field revealed that there are no figures on the extent for most countries, even in the Western world, where the data availability is usually better [55]. One particular difficulty lies in the major differences in the exercise of legal representation. As part of a reform of German law, for example, the concept of the best interests of the person was replaced in favour of the will of the person [56] to take into account the concerns arising from the UN CRPD. Guardians are now obliged to follow the wishes of the person being cared for more closely. However, this is unlikely to have any effect on the practice of coercive measures, as first reviews are suggesting [57]. The percentage of people under guardianship remains particularly high in Germany. According to a publication by the German government, 1.5 percent of the adult population was under legal guardianship in 2015 [58]. It is particularly worrying that 15 percent of these people are unable to exercise their rights at all (German: *Einwilligungsvorbehalt*). For a large proportion of these people, this is due to a psychiatric diagnosis.

Many of these people live in a "special form of accommodation", as inpatient facilities (care homes, outpatient residential group settings, etc.) are called today. In Germany, there were a total of 194,000 people in 2020, 55,800 of whom were people with a "mental disability" ([59]; own calculations). The number of places in residential homes has been increasing internationally for a long period of time [51, 60]. What has rarely been investigated internationally, however, is the number of people who are placed in such residential settings against their will. It is also unclear how many closed residential care places are actually provided for people with psychosocial problems. In Germany, approximately 10 percent of all places in a psychiatric residential home are closed [61], and there is a call—particularly from a professional perspective—for significantly more closed places.

According to the results of a comparative study of living conditions in Germany, slightly less than 50 percent of the respondents in the "special form of housing" who took part in this study were unable to decide wholly on their own which form of housing they wanted to live in. However, even in the outpatient setting, not all respondents believed that they could decide their living arrangements independently. Here, the proportion was still 21 percent [62]. These data make it clear that social-administrative coercion is exercised in areas that cannot necessarily be regarded as formal coercion. It is often the authorities or funding organisations that prevent the social situation of affected people from developing further.

This fact also becomes clear when housing preferences are considered. Housing preferences have been relatively well researched. A corresponding meta-analysis that I conducted revealed that more than 80 percent of the people surveyed with a psychosocial problem wanted to live in their own home [63]. Another meta-analysis in which I was involved showed that more than 60 percent of the people surveyed wanted to be employed in the general labour market and not in workshops or day centres [64]. This also raises the question of how many people are denied access to the general labour market against their will. For Western countries such as Germany, it is estimated that less than one percent of eligible people actually have access to evidence-based programmes such as Supported Employment, which are able to make a place in the primary labour market achievable [65].

In summary, it should be noted that psychiatric coercion—unlike political initiatives suggest and affected individuals and professionals aim for—is not decreasing in most countries but rather is increasing. Furthermore, it should have become clear in which hitherto little-known sector of psychiatric care social and administrative coercion is exercised and that this takes place to a considerable extent, even if exact figures are not known.

1.4 Towards a Nondiscriminatory and Non-pejorative Terminology

Throughout this book, I use terms that may be considered unusual in the context of psychiatry and mental health nursing. Instead of "mental illness" and "disability", I refer to "psychosocial problems" unless otherwise stated and justified, and instead of "psychiatric care", I prefer "psychosocial support".

Why do I think this is necessary? In the following chapters, I will explain why coercion in psychiatric care can no longer be justified and what the consequences of "psychiatry without coercion" would be. However, I am convinced that "psychiatry without coercion" can hardly be realised if we have not questioned and, in some way, overcome our conventional concepts of mental illness. Coercion in psychiatric care is based, as will be explained in detail, on the conviction that a psychiatric diagnosis in combination with risk behaviour legitimises measures against a person's will. A diagnosed mental disorder or a comparable condition is therefore a necessary component of legitimisation. However, and this will also be discussed in detail, the existence of a disorder, as it is usually diagnosed today, is increasingly uncertain, especially from a neuroscientific perspective. This means that the definition and identification of a mental disorder are currently increasingly unclear. This also blurs the boundaries between different psychiatric diagnoses and, above all, between the states of disordered/non-disordered or ill/non-ill.

At the same time, I want to express that we need a terminology in psychiatry and mental health nursing that is more inclusive and diverse in the sense that people who may not define themselves as "ill" are taken into account, even if they have support needs that may not be "psychiatric" in the strictest sense. This could be support from peers, i.e. people who are also affected by psychosocial problems. Up to 80 percent of people who have been diagnosed with "schizophrenia" have no corresponding "insight" [66]. I would like to prevent something that is described in medical ethics and epistemology as epistemic injustice [67]. Epistemic injustice can arise when people do not feel that their specific views and knowledge are adequately recognised, for example, or when people with psychosocial problems are labelled "disabled" or "ill" against their will. Other areas where epistemic injustices have been identified include gender issues or ethnic minorities, who have been discriminated against linguistically and otherwise.

Language, and written language in particular, can be politically charged, as we have learned in recent years in connection with the discussion about gendered language. Even if women were "included" in male terms in certain languages, this was not enough for many women to feel adequately represented. The same applies to terms related to illness, disability or impairment. Just as purely masculine language can be perceived as sexist, terminology that refers to psychosocial problems as "disabled" is in danger of encouraging "ableism", as already mentioned. *Ableism* refers to discrimination against people who cannot fulfil certain ability norms [68].

Even longer than *ableism*, the term *sanism* has been used to describe discrimination in connection with (mental) illness [69]. The starting point for this analysis in the early 1990s was stereotypes used in legal proceedings and articles, for example, that people with psychosocial problems were "weak", "lazy", "sexually uncontrollable", "dangerous" and fundamentally unable to manage their affairs autonomously.

In scientific texts or specialist books, we are also constantly exposed to the danger of using *dismissive* or *sanitised language* [70]. It has long been known from psychiatric stigma research, for example, what consequences this can have for the people affected. According to the sociologist Erving Goffman, in his seminal work on the subject, a person to whom we ascribe a stigma is not regarded as a person of equal value [71]. As Goffman described in detail in the 1960s, this has a massive impact on life and social identity. Therefore, when we speak of "mentally ill people" instead of "people with psychosocial problems", we reduce the identity of these people by making their humanity disappear, and we also do not care about the question of whether the people see themselves as ill. In this respect, we devalue and assign a certain characteristic to the person concerned, which can be humiliating. However, this can also be seen quite differently by the people concerned, as will become clear in a moment.

Of course, as Goffman also described at the time, we generally do not use these terms with the intention of stigmatising. In addition, in medical or nursing professions in particular, it is actually our idea that we want to be supportive with our actions and language. Nevertheless, we have to deal with perspectives that may experience this differently. In addition, for some years now, we have had to deal with activists who expect us professionals to use the language more carefully. In this respect, it is an advantage if the people concerned communicate clearly which terms are more appropriate and which are not. The first guidelines on how researchers can avoid using ableist language have already been published [72], and I try to follow them as closely as possible.

However, such orientations are neither easy to implement nor uncontroversial. We live in sociodiversity, as explained in Chap. 6, and in such a society, there are very different and sometimes contradictory experiences and attitudes towards the terms commonly used in the psychiatric field. I referred above to the now common term "people with… problems". This terminology, which is referred to as *person-first language*, was assumed to be less stigmatising, as it focuses on the person and not the problem [73]. However, this does not necessarily have to be the case, as is communicated mainly by the autism movement. There, an *identity-first language* is favoured in the sense of the neurodiversity terminology [74]. Instead of "people with autism", "autistic people" is expected. The reasoning: Autism is not a deficit that should be less stigmatised but rather an identity with positive connotations, something autistic people can be proud of. Like *identity first* instead of *person first*, terms such as "comorbid" should be replaced by "co-occurring", "symptoms" by "experiences" and "treatment" by "support" [75].

As one can expect, there is resistance to this obvious de-medicalisation of language and normalisation of the phenomena, particularly from parents' associations of autistic people. The argument: Since autism spectrum disorder is a defined clinical condition in the classifications of psychiatry, it must be possible to speak "scientifically accurately" about these disorders and, above all, about the massive limitations, disabilities and deficits of the people affected [76]. As much as I can understand this demand from the parents' point of view, it is not very helpful for the issue under discussion here. From a scientific and epistemological perspective, however, which aims to discuss the significance of "illness" in connection with coercion in psychiatry, it is expedient to *avoid ableism* and *sanism* as much as possible.

At the beginning of this book, as already mentioned, basic terminological definitions should therefore be made. To ensure that a terminology that enables inclusion and diversity is used without prior discrimination or devaluation, the term "psychological phenomenon" should first be defined. A psychological phenomenon describes what every person experiences of themselves at any given time, for example, being in a bad mood or, on the contrary, being completely happy. However, such a state can also mean hearing voices or a strong desire to consume drugs. Importantly, in this context, no judgement is associated with this state. A phenomenon is not necessarily a problem.

However, a psychological condition can result in a "psychosocial problem". The "psychosocial problem" is the second term that I would like to introduce here. A psychosocial problem can arise when the person in question experiences negative consequences from the condition, such as suffering. However, it can also be—and this is why we are not just talking about psychological but psychosocial consequences—a social consequence associated with the phenomenon, for example, the separation of a partner or the loss of a job. Finally, other people can be affected in a social sense, for example, through aggressive behaviour or threats to children's welfare. When psychosocial support systems address psychological phenomena, they are, by definition, problems that have been recognised somewhere and have led to support systems being called in.

I realise that the term "problem" can in some ways have negative connotations that can be interpreted in terms of *ableism* or *sanism*. Not everyone involved necessarily has to subscribe to the view of the problem; as we know, this is how many conflicts arise in psychiatric settings. As I said, my aim is to avoid these connotations as much as possible, which will not always be possible. The difficulty is inherent because support systems such as psychiatric services currently have the power to define what is a problem and what is not. Bearing these difficulties in mind, I use the term "psychosocial problem" as an extension or umbrella term for "mental disorder" or "illness". In Chap. 6, all the facts of the phenomena and problems are described in more detail.

The third term I would like to introduce is "psychosocial support". This is intended to describe any form that people with a psychosocial problem experience as a potential help or solution. As an extension of "psychiatric care", this also includes nonmedical support such as coaching (e.g. job coaching) or peer support from people who are also affected by psychosocial problems. However, conventional treatment and therapy procedures can also be categorised as psychosocial support.

These terms should be used as much as possible. Conventional terminology such as disease, disorder or care will be applied to existing situations and, if they are critically scrutinised, placed in inverted commas.

1.5 The Plan of the Book

The first part of this book aims to show that psychiatric coercion can no longer be justified. At the beginning, Chap. 2 identifies the legitimisation problems for psychiatry. This is followed in Chap. 3 by a reconstruction of the current justification of coercion in psychiatry. Chapters 4 and 5 use research literature to justify that the ethical and legal conditions for the use of coercion do not hold up in light of research.

The second part will then show ways of overcoming coercion in psychiatry. My assumption is that this can be achieved only through fundamental changes to the concept of illness in psychiatry; this is described in Chap. 6. In addition, relevant changes in the support of people with psychosocial problems will be necessary to overcome coercion, as analysed in Chap. 7. Chapter 8 highlights the possible consequences of not using psychiatric interventions against people's will, which can lead to numerous dilemmas. In the concluding epilogue in Chap. 9, I will venture an outlook on further developments, which—this much I can already reveal—will not be particularly optimistic.

References

1. Bull P, Gadsby J, Williams S. Our apology. In: Bull P, Gadsby J, Williams S, editors. Critical mental health nursing: observations from the inside. Monmouth: PCCS Books; 2018. p. VII–X.
2. Lidz CW. Coercion in psychiatric care: what have we learned from research? J Am Acad Psychiatry Law. 1998;26(4):631–7.
3. Szasz T. The case against psychiatric coercion. Indep Rev. 1997;1(4):485–98.
4. Szasz T. Coercion as cure: a critical history of psychiatry. London: Routledge; 2007.
5. Schramme T. Szasz's legacy and current challenges in psychiatry. In: Haldipur CV, Knoll JL, v.d. Luft E, editors. Thomas Szasz: An appraisal of his legacy. Oxford: Oxford UP; 2019. p. 256–71.
6. Scull A. Madness in civilization: a cultural history of insanity from the bible to Freud, from the madhouse to modern medicine. Princeton UP: Princeton; 2015.
7. United Nations. UN convention on the rights of persons with disabilities. 2006. Available from: https://www.un.org/development/desa/disabilities/convention-on-the-rights-of-persons-with-disabilities/convention-on-the-rights-of-persons-with-disabilities-2.html.
8. Della Fina V, Cera R, Palmisano G, editors. The United Nations convention on the rights of persons with disabilities: a commentary. Cham: Springer; 2017.
9. UN General Assembly. Report of the special rapporteur on torture and other cruel, inhuman or degrading treatment or punishment, Juan E Méndez 2013. Contract No.: A/HRC/22/53.
10. Freeman MC, Kolappa K, de Almeida JM, Kleinman A, Makhashvili N, Phakathi S, et al. Reversing hard won victories in the name of human rights: a critique of the general comment on article 12 of the UN convention on the rights of persons with disabilities. Lancet Psychiatry. 2015;2(9):844–50.
11. Gooding P, McSherry B, Roper C. Preventing and reducing 'coercion' in mental health services: an international scoping review of English-language studies. Acta Psychiatr Scand. 2020;142(1):27–39.
12. Allison R, Flemming K. Mental health patients' experiences of softer coercion and its effects on their interactions with practitioners: a qualitative evidence synthesis. J Adv Nurs. 2019;75(11):2274–84.
13. Hotzy F, Jaeger M. Clinical relevance of informal coercion in psychiatric treatment—a systematic review. Front Psych. 2016;7:197.

14. BBC. 'Toxic culture' of abuse at mental health hospital revealed by BBC secret filming. 2022. Available from: https://www.bbc.com/news/uk-63045298.
15. Berlin I. Two concepts of liberty. In: Berlin I, editor. Four essays on liberty. Oxford: Oxford UP; 1969. p. 118–72.
16. Eka IAR, Daulima NHC, Susanti H. The role of informal leaders in restraint and confining people with mental health issues in Manggarai. Indonesia Europ J Mental Health. 2022;17(1):25–36.
17. Gupta DK, Verma KK, Baniya GC, Chaurotia V, Sidana R, Khandelwal SK. Road to freedom: experiences of unfettering and rehabilitating chained mentally ill persons in rural India. World Soc Psych. 2024;6(3):137–45.
18. Thumiger C. Ancient greek and roman traditions. In: Eghigian G, editor. The Routledge history of madness and mental health. London: Routledge; 2017. p. 42–61.
19. Hempeler C, Braun E, Potthoff S, Gather J, Scholten M. When treatment pressures become coercive: a context-sensitive model of informal coercion in mental healthcare. Am J Bioeth. 2024;24(12):74–86.
20. Richter D. Treatment pressure: a step forward, but not the final word on "informal coercion". Am J Bioeth. 2024;24(12):113–4.
21. Goltz SM. An analysis of types and targets of coercive interference. J Theor Philos Psychol. 2024;44(1):42–58.
22. Savage MK, Lepping P, Newton-Howes G, Arnold R, Staggs VS, Kisely S, et al. Comparison of coercive practices in worldwide mental healthcare: overcoming difficulties resulting from variations in monitoring strategies. BJPsych Open. 2024;10(1):e26.
23. Sheridan Rains L, Zenina T, Dias MC, Jones R, Jeffreys S, Branthonne-Foster S, et al. Variations in patterns of involuntary hospitalisation and in legal frameworks: an international comparative study. Lancet Psychiatry. 2019;6(5):403–17.
24. Fornazari C, Canfield M, Laranjeira R. Real world evidence in involuntary psychiatric hospitalizations: 64,685 cases. Brazilian J Psychiatry. 2022;44(3):308–11.
25. Di Lorenzo R, Reami M, Dragone D, Morgante M, Panini G, Rovesti S, et al. Involuntary hospitalizations in an Italian acute psychiatric Ward: a 6-year retrospective analysis. Patient Prefer Adherence. 2023;17:3403–20.
26. Kalanj K, Ćurković M, Peček M, Orešković S, Orbanić A, Marshall R. Impact of the COVID-19 pandemic on acute mental health admissions in Croatia. Frontiers. Public Health. 2023;11:11.
27. Richter D, Rühle Andersson S, Burr C, Domonell K, Melina H, Hegedüs A, et al. Menschenrechte in der schweizerischen Psychiatrie - Zum Stand der Umsetzung der UN-BRK. Psychiatrische Pflege. 2023;8(2):9–12.
28. Lebenbaum M, Chiu M, Vigod S, Kurdyak P. Prevalence and predictors of involuntary psychiatric hospital admissions in Ontario, Canada: a population-based linked administrative database study. BJPsych Open. 2018;4(2):31–8.
29. Goulet M-H, Cassivi C, Hupé C, Jean-Baptiste F, Dumais A. Seclusion and mechanical restraint in the wake of the COVID-19 pandemic: an increased use in mental health settings. Front Psychiatry. 2024;15:15.
30. Loyal JP, Lavergne MR, Shirmaleki M, Fischer B, Kaoser R, Makolewksi J, et al. Trends in involuntary psychiatric hospitalization in British Columbia: descriptive analysis of population-based linked administrative data from 2008 to 2018. Can J Psychiatry. 2023;68(4):257–68.
31. Wild K, Sawhney J, Wyder M, Sebar B, Gill N. Reasons behind the rise in involuntary psychiatric treatment under mental health act 2016, Queensland, Australia—clinician perspectives. Int J Law Psychiatry. 2025;98:102061.
32. Sheridan Rains L, Weich S, Maddock C, Smith S, Keown P, Crepaz-Keay D, et al. Understanding increasing rates of psychiatric hospital detentions in England: development and preliminary testing of an explanatory model. BJPsych Open. 2020;6(5):e88.
33. Hill SA, Riordan-Eva E, Hosking A. Trends in the number of restricted patients in England and Wales 2003–2016: implications for forensic psychiatry services. Med Sci Law. 2019;59(1):42–8.

References

34. Keown P, Murphy H, McKenna D, McKinnon I. Changes in the use of the mental health act 1983 in England 1984/85 to 2015/16. Br J Psychiatry. 2018;213(4):595–9.
35. Schölin L, Borschmann R, Chopra A. Temporal patterns and individual characteristics of compulsory treatment orders for mental disorders in Scotland from 2007 to 2020. BJPsych Open. 2024;10(6):e204.
36. Steinert T, Salize H, Dreßing H, Juckel G, Steinhart I. ZIPHER: Zwangsmaßnahmen Im Psychiatrischen Hilfesystem: Erfassung und Reduktion. Bundesministerium für Gesundheitswesen. 2022.
37. Flammer E, Eisele F, Hirsch S, Steinert T. Increase in coercive measures in psychiatric hospitals in Germany during the COVID-19 pandemic. PLoS One. 2022;17(8):e0264046.
38. Vruwink FJ, Wierdsma A, Noorthoorn EO, Nijman HLI, Mulder CL. Number of seclusions in The Netherlands higher in the 7 years since the end of a Nationwide seclusion-reduction program. Frontiers. Psychiatry. 2021;12:12.
39. Lee G, Cohen D. Incidences of involuntary psychiatric detentions in 25 U.S. States Psychiatric Serv. 2021;72(1):61–8.
40. Yang Y, Li W, An F-R, Wang Y-Y, Ungvari GS, Balbuena L, et al. Voluntary and involuntary admissions for severe mental illness in China: a systematic review and meta-analysis. Psychiatr Serv. 2020;71(1):83–6.
41. Välimäki M, Yang M, Vahlberg T, Lantta T, Pekurinen V, Anttila M, et al. Trends in the use of coercive measures in Finnish psychiatric hospitals: a register analysis of the past two decades. BMC Psychiatry. 2019;19(1):230.
42. Ministry of Health. Office of the Director of mental health and addiction services: regulatory report 1 July 2021 to 30 June 2022. Wellington: Ministry Health; 2023.
43. Lucey JV, Kiernan G, Farrelly J, Downey A, Stepala P. Use of restrictive practices in approved mental health centres in Ireland: consideration of five years of national data. Ir J Psychol Med. 2024;1-6:15.
44. Hansen TE, Bloom JD, Blekic A. The dramatic decline of civil commitment in Oregon, 1972 to 2020. J Am Acad Psychiatry Law Online. 2022;50(4):533–40.
45. Lickiewicz J, Efkemann SA, Husum TL, Lantta T, Pingani L, Whittington R. Expert opinions on improving coercion data collection across Europe: a concept mapping study. Frontiers. Psychiatry. 2024;15:15.
46. Smith A, van Voren R, Liebrenz M. Resurgent trends in punitive psychiatry in The Russian Federation. The lancet regional health—Europe 2024;42, 42.
47. Rzhevskaya N. Restriction of the rights and coercion of patients in a psychiatric hospital: the opinion of people with mental disorders and psychiatrists. Iran Rehabil J. 2023;21(3):533–42.
48. Jay M, Mahdanian AA, Tavakoli E, Puras D. Political abuse of Iranian psychiatry and psychiatric services. Lancet. 2022;400(10367):1923–4.
49. Koh KA, Gorman BL. Reimagining institutionalization and a continuum of Care for People Experiencing Homelessness and Mental Illness. JAMA. 2023;329(17):1449–50.
50. Mikellides G, Stefani A, Tantele M. Community treatment orders: international perspective. BJPsych Int. 2019;16(4):83–6.
51. Chow WS, Priebe S. How has the extent of institutional mental healthcare changed in Western Europe? Analysis of data since 1990. BMJ Open. 2016;6(4):e010188.
52. Traub H-J, Ross T. Ein Revival der "Forensifizierung"? Recht und Psychiatrie. 2023;41(3):150–9.
53. Tomlin J, Lega I, Braun P, Kennedy HG, Herrando VT, Barroso R, et al. Forensic mental health in Europe: some key figures. Soc Psychiatry Psychiatr Epidemiol. 2021;56(1):109–17.
54. Beis P, Graf M, Hachtel H. Impact of legal traditions on forensic mental health treatment worldwide. Front Psych. 2022;13:876619.
55. Office of the Public Advocate. Guardianship around the world – a resource on international adult guardianship systems. World Congress on Adult Guardianship, Guardianship and the United Nations Disabilities Convention; 2012.

56. Braun E, Gather J, Henking T, Vollmann J, Scholten M. Das Verständnis von Wohl im Betreuungsrecht—eine Analyse anlässlich der Streichung des Wohlbegriffs aus dem reformierten Gesetz. Ethik Med. 2022;34(4):515–28.
57. Henking T. Die Reform des Betreuungsrechts. Nervenarzt. 2022;93(11):1125–33.
58. Bundesministerium der Justiz und für Verbraucherschutz (BMJV). Qualität in der rechtlichen Betreuung – Abschlussbericht. Köln. 2018.
59. BAGÜS. BAGÜS Kennzahlenvergleich Eingliederungshilfe 2022 – Berichtsjahr 2020. Münster: Bundesarbeitsgemeinschaft der überörtlichen Träger der Sozialhilfe und der Eingliederungshilfe. 2022.
60. Priebe S, Badesconyi A, Fioritti A, Hansson L, Kilian R, Torres-Gonzales F, et al. Reinstitutionalisation in mental health care: comparison of data on service provision from six European countries. Br Med J. 2005;330(7483):123–6.
61. Steinhart I, Jenderny S, Wassiliwizky M, Heinz A. Personenzentrierte Hilfen, aber geschlossen untergebracht? Zur Situation der geschlossenen Heime in Deutschland. Nervenarzt. 2021;92(9):941–7.
62. Wienberg G, Steinhart I. Wirksamkeit der Eingliederungshilfe Wohnen für Menschen mit seelischen Behinderungen in Nordrhein-Westfalen—Projekt WiEWohnen NRW. Bielefeld: Bethel Regional; n.d.
63. Richter D, Hoffmann H. Preference for independent housing of persons with mental disorders: systematic review and meta-analysis. Admin Pol Ment Health. 2017;44(6):817–23.
64. Adamus C, Richter D, Sutor K, Zürcher SJ, Mötteli S. Preference for competitive employment in people with mental disorders: a systematic review and meta-analysis of proportions. J Occup Rehabil. 2024;35:143.
65. Jäckel D, Nischk D. Warum tun wir eigentlich nicht, was wir schon wissen? Zum Stand der Supported Employment-Implementierung in Deutschland. Sozialpsychiatrische Informationen. 2024:20–32.
66. Lincoln TM, Lullmann E, Rief W. Correlates and long-term consequences of poor insight in patients with schizophrenia. Sys Rev Schizophrenia Bullet. 2007;33(6):1324–42.
67. Fricker M. Epistemic injustice: power and the ethics of knowing. Oxford: Oxford University Press; 2007.
68. Buchner T, Pfahl L, Traue B. Zur Kritik der Fähigkeiten: Ableism als neue Forschungsperspektive der Disability Studies und ihrer Partner_innen. Zeitschrift für Inklusion. 2015;0(2)
69. Perlin ML. On Sanism. SMU Law. Review. 1992;46:373–408.
70. Poole JM, Jivraj T, Arslanian A, Bellows K, Chiasson S, Hakimy H, et al. Sanism, 'mental health', and social work/education: A review and call to action. Intersectionalities 2012;1:20–36.
71. Goffman E. Stigma: notes on the Management of Spoiled Identity. Englewood Cliffs, NJ: Prentice Hall; 1963.
72. Bottema-Beutel K, Kapp SK, Lester JN, Sasson NJ, Hand BN. Avoiding ableist language: suggestions for autism researchers. Autism Adulthood. 2021;3(1):18–29.
73. Volkow ND, Gordon JA, Koob GF. Choosing appropriate language to reduce the stigma around mental illness and substance use disorders. Neuropsychopharmacology. 2021;46(13):2230–2.
74. Keating CT, Hickman L, Leung J, Monk R, Montgomery A, Heath H, et al. Autism-related language preferences of English-speaking individuals across the globe: a mixed methods investigation. Autism. Research. 2022;
75. Monk R, Whitehouse AJO, Waddington H. The use of language in autism research. Trends Neurosci. 2022;45(11):791–3.
76. Singer A, Lutz A, Escher J, Halladay A. A full semantic toolbox is essential for autism research and practice to thrive. Autism. Research. 2022;16:1–5.

Human Rights and Psychiatric Coercion: The Legitimisation Problem for (Social) Psychiatry

2.1 Introduction

Under what circumstances is it professionally, legally and ethically legitimate to restrict the rights of people with psychosocial problems and subject them to various forms of coercion? Such restrictions and coercive measures, which are to be understood as human rights violations according to the United Nations Convention on the Rights of Persons with Disabilities (hereinafter: UN CRPD), take place, for example, when those affected are denied the right to live in their own home on the grounds of an illness and its consequences, when they are assigned a sheltered workshop place instead of support in the primary labour market or when they are taken to a psychiatric hospital and treated against their will.

In almost all countries, there is also the instrument of legal representation, i.e. the possibility of people (commonly called "guardians") taking over certain matters for people with severe psychosocial problems. Legal or statutory representation against the will is a massive social exclusion from the legal system, which is usually encouraged or advocated by mental health services or staff.

With respect to the legitimacy of such restrictions, a bitter dispute has recently arisen between representatives of psychiatric care on the one hand and representatives of affected groups as well as legal and political experts on the other hand. In the view of the United Nations, such a restriction should be fundamentally questioned. "(T)he will and preferences of the person concerned…" must always be taken into account in regard to measures relating to human rights standards for people with disabilities. This is stated in Article 12 of the UN CRPD from 2006 [1]. In other words, according to this position, human rights and individual freedom may be restricted only to the extent that this is possible in accordance with the will and preferences of the person affected by the measure. The entire article and this passage have proven to be among the most controversial legal passages in the recent history of psychiatry. The term "disability" stands—in my view not very happily—in the UN publications for various limitations that people can experience, including people with "psychosocial disabilities", as it says there.

The convention thus clearly goes beyond the standard that usually prevails in medicine. Respecting the person's will and preferences is not the same as acting "in the person's interest" or "for the person's benefit", as is still customary in medicine, for example, when treating unconscious accident victims. In the case of actions in the person's best interest, a medical decision is made on the basis of assumptions without actually inquiring about the person's wishes and preferences. Depending on the situation, this is often not possible in any other way.

During the COVID-19 pandemic, however, we have had to learn in many different ways that fundamental rights and freedoms can and must be restricted for medical reasons. Without quarantine and lockdown measures, there would have been significantly more cases of illness and death. The relevant empirical research on this topic has impressively confirmed this [2]. The restriction of human rights/freedoms/fundamental rights for medical reasons can therefore be legitimised professionally, ethically and legally because they are often not only in the public interest but also, from a medical point of view, in the interest of the people affected by the measures, even if they do not correspond to their will.

This also applies in a similar way to restrictions on personal freedoms imposed by psychiatry. According to conventional psychiatric justification, there are medical reasons for taking measures against a person's will, such as forced hospitalisation, seclusion/isolation or restraint, as well as detention in a forensic hospital following a criminal offence. If the person is mentally ill in the broadest sense, if they are incapable of judgement, if the intervention against the will of the person concerned does more good than harm and if it is in the person's best interests, then it is justifiable [3]. This justification is based on the four main principles of ethics established in medicine, namely, the principle of *beneficence*, the principle of *non-maleficence*, respect for the *autonomy* of the person concerned and *justice* [4].

A medical measure against the will of the person concerned may therefore be carried out both in an epidemic situation and in the context of psychiatric treatment for ethical and legal reasons if the following criteria are met:

1. It is a defined disease.
2. The disease must have a relatively serious impact on the person affected, on other people or on the population.
3. Effective therapeutic interventions are available.
4. The measure must be for the overall benefit of the person and must not harm them (e.g. as a side effect).
5. The application must be proportionate.
6. Freedoms must be restricted as little as possible.

This is much like the conventional justification for restricting civil liberties on medical grounds. In recent years, psychiatry, which essentially represents this position in connection with coercion in treatment, has had to address criticism from unexpected quarters. First, the United Nations and its suborganisations, such as the

2.1 Introduction

World Health Organisation (WHO), have repeatedly drawn attention to the aspects of violated human rights, such as those arising from coercive measures. In an additional commentary on Article 12 of the UN CRPD, the responsible UN committee explained that, contrary to the legal traditions of many countries, the article calls for the separation of mental capacity and legal capacity [5]. This means that people who are certified as lacking mental capacity should be allowed to refuse medical treatment and thus also coercive psychiatric measures, as they retain their legal capacity in principle. The instrument of legal representation (e.g. guardianship) would thus become obsolete, at least if it were to happen against the will of the person concerned.

Second, various UN rapporteurs have repeatedly pointed out the violation of the rights of people with psychosocial problems and denounced coercive measures such as restraint, seclusion/isolation and forced medication. The controversial demand in psychiatric circles is that coercive measures should be abolished as a matter of principle. The disputes between the psychiatric associations and the suborganisations of the United Nations reached a temporary climax when the UN Human Rights Council appointed a rapporteur to deal with torture, abuse and degrading treatment in medical institutions [6]. Psychiatric institutions were particularly affected by this report, as it called for the revision of legal regulations that allow coercive measures in general: "Legislation authorizing the institutionalization of persons with disabilities on the grounds of their disability without their free and informed consent must be abolished". In addition, the main report established a particular link between coercion and the conventional biomedical paradigm in psychiatry. Accordingly, the report calls for a fundamental change: "Coercion, medicalization and exclusion, which are vestiges of traditional psychiatric care relationships, must be replaced with a modern understanding of recovery and evidence-based services that restore dignity and return rights holders to their families and communities" [7: 18].

Third, the World Health Organisation (WHO) recently published new guidelines for psychiatric care that focus on the avoidance of coercion and call for human rights to be respected in psychiatry. Here, too, a departure from the biomedical and primarily medication-based paradigm is called for. The guidelines explicitly expect WHO member states to ensure the right of affected people to refuse any form of psychiatric intervention [8].

The circumstances described by the UN organisations were not compatible with the traditional medico-psychiatric self-image. Furthermore, different ethical judgements regarding the importance of human rights can also be assumed. While the UN CRPD and various other UN documents ascribe a prominent position to human rights and civil liberties, this is not the case according to the current standard work on biomedical ethics. It states that "…human rights are no more fundamental than moral virtues in a universal morality…" [4, p. 4]. In other words, human rights are no more important than, for example, professional medical ethics.

For these reasons, there have been few relevant changes in the core area of mental health care to date. At best, there have been legal changes in some countries in the nonmedical area of support for people with disabilities, which can certainly be seen as being in line with the UN CRPD. The extent to which this has actually improved the situation of the people concerned remains to be seen in future evaluations.

However, it was not only conventional biomedically orientated psychiatry that had problems with this criticism and the associated demand for the abolition of measures against the will of the person concerned. One might have expected social psychiatry to adopt these demands and initiatives. Although this is happening to a limited extent, the reactions of many professionals are different—among nurses, too [9]. The general demand for the abolition of coercion in psychiatry is highly controversial even within social psychiatry, as I will show in detail in the following section.

The conflict mentioned at the beginning between those who want to abolish coercion and those who want to retain coercion as a last but indispensable means can, in my opinion, be resolved, as I hope to be able to explain in the course of the book. To this point, we have basically only been talking about the abolition of measures against a person's will in the context of care and support. However, I am convinced that the UN CRPD and related initiatives such as "QualityRights" [10] can also be read as a guide for the implementation of contemporary psychiatry in the sense of psychosocial support. In the following section, the various topics addressed by the Convention are presented in more detail: which human rights violations are meant, and what would be the consequences of consistent implementation?

The first important thing to understand about the Convention on the Rights of Persons with Disabilities is that it does not apply only to people with mental or psychosocial problems. The Convention applies to people with any form of disability, i.e. both physical and other problems. The central requirement of the Convention is the nondiscrimination of people with disabilities. People with disabilities should be treated in the same way as people without disabilities. They should enjoy the same rights as all other people, and this also applies to their rights in the healthcare system.

Later in the book, as indicated earlier, I will discuss the terminology used here, in particular why the terminology of "disability" is not useful in my view and why a neutral and inclusive term such as "psychosocial problems" seems more appropriate. In the following section, however, I follow the official terminology of the Convention to avoid misunderstandings.

2.2 Human Rights and the Social Model of Disability

Article 1 of the UN CRPD describes how disabilities should be understood, namely, "interaction with various barriers [that] may hinder their full and effective participation in society on an equal basis with others". This means that the concept of disability follows the so-called social model [11], in which the problem no longer lies primarily in the person, as was the case in earlier medical models. Previously, the person had to adapt to an environment of some kind, for example, by choosing the living situation according to the person's possibilities and skills. As a rule, no further development then took place. On the other hand, concepts such as "residential coaching" provide support services that help people cope with housing situations that were previously considered impossible for them. In other words, the problem of disability arises in interaction with the social environment, and the environment must be adapted to the person in such a way that the person can ideally live according to their preferences.

Figure 2.1 summarises the key features and implications of both the medical model and the social model of disability (see also [12]). As already indicated, the medical model of disability assumes that disability is a characteristic of the person. The person *is* disabled. Disabled people can integrate by adapting to their environmental conditions. If this is not possible, they are supported in special institutions such as homes or workshops. In contrast, the social model of disability is based on the decisive reasons in the person's environment. A person becomes disabled because the social environment does not respond flexibly enough to the person's needs. In contrast to social integration, inclusion takes place here by adapting the social environment to the person.

Behind the entire Convention is the aspiration to "enable persons with disabilities to live independently and participate fully in all aspects of life", as Article 9 states. This means the full inclusion of people in society and the opportunity to achieve everything that people without disabilities can achieve.

Consequently, full participation also means legal equality. The already mentioned, highly controversial Article 12 demands that people with disabilities retain their legal capacity and, if necessary, receive support to exercise their rights. This article is generally interpreted to mean that legal representation against the person's will is no longer permitted. These are to be replaced by supported decision-making, which should essentially consider the person's will and preferences.

Article 15, sentence 1 of the UN CRPD reads: "No one shall be subjected to torture or to cruel, inhuman or degrading treatment or punishment. In particular, no one shall be subjected without his or her free consent to medical or scientific experimentation". This sentence defines involuntary detention and treatment as close to or—as in various UN publications—as torture and degradation. It follows that any

Medical model	Social model
The reason for the disability lies in the person	The reason for the disability lies in the social environment, which does not react flexibly enough to the needs of the person concerned
→ The person is disabled	→ The person becomes disabled
Adaptation of the person concerned to the environment or care in a special institution	Primary adaptation of the environment to the needs of the person concerned; no care in a special institution
→ Integration	→ Inclusion

Fig. 2.1 Medical and social model of disability

involuntary form of medical intervention in connection with disability must be avoided. Treatment in psychiatric settings must therefore be exclusively voluntary. While a negative formulation is used here, Article 25, which describes access to healthcare services, explicitly states that states undertake "…to provide care of the same quality to persons with disabilities as to others, including on the basis of free and informed consent…".

The independent living of persons with disabilities is set out in Article 19. It states, among other things, that "(p)ersons with disabilities have the opportunity to choose their place of residence and where and with whom they live on an equal basis with others and are not obliged to live in a particular living arrangement (…)". They shall have access to support services, "including personal assistance necessary to support living and inclusion in the community, and to prevent isolation or segregation from the community". This is intended to emphasise that people with disabilities should no longer have their living arrangements dictated to them but should live as they wish and receive the necessary assistance. Placements against their will in care homes or similar settings would therefore no longer be permitted. In this context, Article 25 calls for nationwide outpatient care, including in rural areas, with regard to healthcare services.

According to the Convention, independent living and full participation also includes equal access to educational opportunities. Article 24 regulates inclusive education, which is intended to prevent the segregation of programmes for people with and without disabilities. Building on the education article, Article 27 formulates the right to "the opportunity to gain a living by work freely chosen or accepted in a labour market and work environment that is open, inclusive and accessible to persons with disabilities", "including equal opportunities and equal remuneration for work of equal value". Employment in sheltered workshops is therefore not equivalent, and people with disabilities must first be given access to the general labour market if they want to. Finally, Article 28 formulates the right to an adequate standard of living "for themselves and their families, including adequate food, clothing and housing, and to the continuous improvement of living conditions".

If we summarise the articles of the Convention just mentioned, which are particularly relevant for people with psychosocial problems, we can derive clear mandates for psychiatry in general and for social psychiatry in particular. People with psychosocial problems should live, work and be supported in the way they wish. Mental health support in this sense would mean [1] exclusively voluntary treatment, [2] supported forms of living according to the person's preference, [3] ensuring education and vocational training, [4] ensuring access to the general labour market, [5] preventing poverty, and [6] new forms of decision-making that prioritise the person's will and preferences.

In principle, most professionals in psychiatric or psychosocial care are in agreement with the above-mentioned mandates. However, I would like to use two current controversies to show that this agreement has clear limits and that, when push comes to shove, the principles no longer apply. The first is the issue of coercion and therapy, which has already been mentioned, and the second is assisted suicide or medical aid in dying for people with psychosocial problems, i.e. the coercion to live that prevails in most countries of the world.

2.3 The Controversy Surrounding the Use of Coercion in Social Psychiatry

As mentioned above, the use of coercion in mental health care is highly controversial. The controversy continues to take place in various areas of psychiatry, unfortunately only rarely in mental health nursing. With a few exceptions [13, 14], aspects such as the UN CRPD and its implications are rarely discussed. For this reason, the discussion in social psychiatry is traced here.

Recently, the controversy surrounding coercion in treatment has been discussed in various German- and English-language psychiatry journals. On the one hand, they were leading figures from the social psychiatry community; on the other hand, they were equally well-known professionals as well as representatives of those affected. The subject of the controversy was the question of whether psychiatric care can fundamentally do without coercion and what consequences such a renunciation would entail.

This topic and the associated controversies are not new. In the early 1960s, the US psychiatrist and psychoanalyst Thomas Szasz concluded, "There is no medical, moral or legal justification for involuntary psychiatric interventions. These are crimes against humanity" [15: 268]. The reason for this conclusion was as simple as it was controversial: In Szasz's view, the idea of mental illness was a "myth". Mental illness had been "invented" by psychiatry, deviating from the central insights of medicine. In contrast to physical illnesses, which are based on demonstrable changes to the body structure (e.g. a tumour or a fracture), a new criterion was introduced in the case of psychiatry, that is, functional change. According to Szasz, however, functionally explained diseases are not "real" diseases, as they were not discovered but invented.

However, what should happen to people who have committed a serious norm violation, such as a criminal offense, against the background of a supposed mental illness? Here too, Szasz's answer was as simple as it was controversial: These people should be imprisoned. "Institutions of a punitive nature (prisons) should house those whom society wishes to segregate. The primary purpose of this institution should be the establishment of public safety" [16: 170]. People who were considered mentally ill were, in Szasz's opinion, nothing more than Jews or non-white people, who at various points in history were declared scapegoats.

Thomas Szasz, who, together with the British psychiatrist R.D. Laing, the American sociologist Erving Goffman and the French philosopher Michel Foucault, is now counted among the founders of "anti-psychiatry", was not fundamentally opposed to psychiatric support for people who voluntarily sought it. According to his interpretation, these people were concerned primarily with questions and uncertainties about how to lead their lives, such as the realisation of life goals. Martin Zinkler and Sebastian von Peter make a very similar argument in their 2019 article

"End Coercion in Mental Health Services—Toward a System Based on Support Only" [17]. They also propose that law enforcement authorities should no longer be able to take people to a psychiatric hospital against their will, as is currently possible. However, their reasoning is different to that of Szasz. Zinkler and von Peter's reform ideas are based on the aforementioned UN CRPD, which prohibits discrimination against people with physical or mental disabilities compared with people without disabilities. Accordingly, people with and without disabilities must be treated equally in principle. "The principle of non-discrimination in the Convention stipulates that persons with an assumed or diagnosed mental illness must not be treated legally different than persons without this attribution" [17: 4].

These considerations do not neglect to support those who refuse hospital treatment. Alternatives include assistance with social problems such as homelessness and poverty, as well as home treatment, i.e. acute psychiatric treatment in the patient's own home. However, this form of psychiatry, conceived exclusively as supportive, is intended to dispense with the traditional "dual function" of treatment and order/control by discarding the control function. The authors hope that this will lead to greater acceptance of psychiatric support services if the users realise that the possibilities for coercive measures can no longer take place in psychiatry but at best in the area of police and criminal law.

The article by Martin Zinkler and Sebastian von Peter provoked harsh reactions. According to psychiatrists Maximilian Gahr and Manfred Spitzer in a rebuttal [18: 136], the considerations are "…in terms of psychiatric history… a step backwards by approximately 200 years…" (Translations from the German have been provided by the author of the book). According to their assessment, the approach of psychiatry operating exclusively without coercion is essentially "…anti-patient, because it can run counter to a person's interest in receiving professional help when they are ill". [18: 137] Psychiatrist Peter Brieger and psychologist Susanne Menzel even characterised the approach as "inhumane" [19: 297]. The principle of exclusively non-coercive psychiatric care inadmissibly emphasises the aspect of self-determination over the principles of care and non-harm.

The psychiatrist Tilman Steinert argued somewhat differently against the ideas of Martin Zinkler and Sebastian von Peter. His central objection relates to the difference between physical and mental illnesses. This is to be seen in the fact "…that mental illnesses affect the organ responsible for a person's volitional decisions, the brain. All mental illnesses can—in a relatively broad sense—be understood as functional disorders of the brain" [20: 30]. Due to this difference, mental illnesses have a special status, as they can restrict the ability to make free-will decisions. Against this background, it is justifiable in principle that medical professionals should be allowed to order measures that restrict freedom in the interests of other people, analogous to infection control measures that can make quarantine mandatory for people with existing mental capacity.

However, the argument that professionals should be allowed to order measures in the interests of people with "mental illnesses" was then drastically contradicted in a statement by two German associations of service users. The view associated with the described approach of psychiatry without coercion reflects "… what those with experience of psychiatry have long criticised about the existing psychiatric system. Those affected regularly draw attention to the fact that psychiatric violence runs counter to the medical principle of non-harm and is considered unethical and inhumane" [21: 36]. The associations objected to what they saw as the instrumentalisation of the benefit of those affected by the critical positions cited above in relation to the concept of psychiatry operating exclusively without coercion. This instrumentalisation was part of the "psychiatric violence" experienced by those affected.

In summary, the perspectives on autonomy, freedom of choice and "mental illness" differ fundamentally. On the one hand, there is the conventional psychiatric and social psychiatry view that an illness impairs the exercise of one's own rights and therefore requires a proxy decision by medical professionals under certain circumstances. On the other hand, those affected dispute that anyone should be allowed to act as a proxy without further ado, regardless of whether the impaired person is considered "mentally ill".

Incidentally, the latter position also corresponds to the views of the United Nations CRPD. Accordingly, mental disabilities must not lead to legal restrictions. This means that substitute decision-making, for example, by a guardian or a legal representative, is basically not permitted. This legal position has triggered considerable debate [22, 23] but also considerable resistance [24] in the psychiatric community.

2.4 The Controversy Surrounding Medical Aid in Dying for People with Psychosocial Problems

The second topic also revolves around the question of the autonomy of people with mental health problems. Apart from the direct issue of coercion already mentioned, no other discussion is likely as emotional as the discussion concerning assisted suicide or medical aid in dying (MAID) for people with psychosocial problems. In various European countries, MAID is also permitted for people with mental health problems, for example, in Switzerland, Belgium and the Netherlands.

However, to be clear from the outset, a ban on MAID is a variant of the administrative or social coercion described in the introduction. People are forced either to continue living with their suffering or to seek an undignified way out, or even one that harms other people. Of course, many readers will not necessarily take note of this section with approval, as MAID has ethical, medical-psychiatric or even religious connotations. I am not primarily concerned here with the question of the permissibility of MAID but with the use of psychiatrically legitimised coercion against people who want to end their lives.

I would therefore like to make two brief comments in advance. For the sake of transparency, it must be reported here that I am involved in this controversy in German-speaking countries and that I am a supporter of MAID for people with psychosocial problems [25, 26]. In the course of a thorough examination of this issue, and this is the second remark, I have drawn terminological consequences for myself that clearly distinguish "suicide" from "MAID". According to the American

Association of Suicidology [27] and German bioethicists [28], suicide is an act in the context of an acute mental disorder, whereas MAID is a well-considered step that does not occur in the context of an acute problem.

From the point of view of many psychiatric professionals, there are various reasons against assisted suicide. First, there is the history of psychiatry, which, with the "euthanasia" of people with mental impairments during the reign of National Socialism, contains a dark chapter that cannot be surpassed. The conceptual history of social psychiatry is—which may surprise some readers—overshadowed by the ideas of racial hygiene [29]. It is therefore all the more understandable that postwar social psychiatry, particularly in Germany, sought to draw a clear dividing line between mental health care and the killing of impaired people. Against this background, Asmus Finzen, one of the best-known reform psychiatrists in Germany and Switzerland, has lamented the fact that Belgium and the Netherlands, for example, have even considered authorising active euthanasia for people with mental illness [30].

Another reason is the medical categorisation of suicidality as a pathological phenomenon. What many psychiatric clinicians today basically take for granted, namely, that suicide predominantly has a psychopathological background, has not always been the case and is still not the case in parts of the world today. For a long time, suicide was a moral, religious and even illegal act that has only recently been medicalised and pathologised [31]. It is well known that one of the central tasks of psychiatric care is to prevent suicide; in almost all legal-psychiatric contexts, suicidal acts are a reason to use coercion against the person concerned and, under certain circumstances, to treat them against their will. This distinguishes psychiatry from other medical disciplines. If a person with severe diabetes mellitus endangers themselves by not adhering to their diet, this usually has no legal consequences.

In addition, according to another explicitly social psychiatry argument against assisted suicide, the possibility of assisted suicide would send out a "devastating signal" if it were to bring mental illness close to incurability, according to sociologist Silvia Krumm, in a pro and con discussion with me [32]. This would destroy any hope of recovery and would result in a life with the illness, which would run counter to the recovery concept promoted in social psychiatry.

From the conventional psychiatric perspective and the social psychiatry perspective, no distinction is usually made between suicide and MAID. A MAID requires a well-considered decision, which is often not the case with suicide. The pathologisation of an act that seeks to bring about one's own death now leads to a circular argument, as suicidal behaviour can be a symptom of a mental disorder. Anyone who wants to end their life is suicidal, and anyone who is suicidal is mentally ill and can therefore lack capacity, according to the abbreviated argument. When clinicians have to assess capacity, as is often the case in the run-up to MAID, "… determining competence is difficult when the wish to die is part of the underlying syndrome itself", according to the influential psychiatrist Paul Appelbaum, who is highly critical of assisted suicide [33: 316].

Once again, it is therefore a question of the autonomous decision of people who have psychosocial problems. If life with these psychosocial problems is experienced as no longer bearable, then both conventional psychiatry and many people in the social psychiatry community deny those affected the right to make an autonomous decision about this step. When the Swiss Academy of Medical Sciences published new guidelines on assisted suicide in healthcare a few years ago, which also included people with mental health problems, large sections of the medical community reacted with drastic rejection. "Any objectivity and any shared subjectivity with regard to the question of whether suffering is unbearable are thus sacrificed on the altar of the principle of autonomy" [34: 911]" When the highest court in Germany, the Federal Constitutional Court, called for new legal principles in dealing with assisted suicide, many clinicians objected because they saw this as a kind of glorification of suicide as a freedom right.

From the perspective of rights for people with disabilities, as set out in the UN CRPD, for example, the exclusion of mental health problems as a cause of suicide is a fundamental form of discrimination. People with physical illnesses are granted MAID, whereas this is not the case for people with profound psychosocial problems. This clearly contradicts the nondiscrimination principle of the UN CRPD. If people with unbearable psychosocial conditions are denied this step as part of a well-considered conclusion, in my opinion, this is not compatible with a recovery perspective of nursing and mental health care. For me, the contradiction is obvious: we promote recovery and empowerment so that people with psychosocial problems can regain control of their lives and the decisions associated with them. Recovery also means taking risks and not ruling out everything that could lead to problematic situations from the outset. This aspect of the recovery process is referred to as "positive risk-taking" [35]. We also want to move away from a paternalistic attitude in social psychiatry and mental health nursing, which suggests that it knows what is good for the person concerned. Ultimately, however, this means that we have to allow the person concerned to make decisions that we do not necessarily like. In the particular case of MAID, this includes the decision not to continue living. It is not acceptable to say take your affairs back into your own hands but only for as long as it suits me.

Furthermore, the illness concept of suicide should not be left as the only possible interpretation. It is possible to commit suicide for rational reasons [36]. Recently, there has been increasing criticism of so-called psychological autopsy studies, which retrospectively search for psychological causes of suicide and find these causes in 70–90 percent of cases. From a methodological point of view, such retrospective studies are highly dubious [37]; interestingly, scientifically adequate studies that are conducted prospectively have not yet found any stable predictors of suicide [38].

From an epidemiological perspective, doubts about an exclusively pathologising perspective are also justified. Social developments, such as the financial crisis at the end of the 2000s, have led to significantly increased suicide rates in Greece [39] and Spain [40]. In German history, the reunification of the two German states, East Germany and West Germany, is, to a certain extent, a natural experiment that suggests an inverse relationship [41]. The suicide rates in the territory of the former GDR were already significantly higher than those in the West before the Second

World War and remained high during the socialist regime. However, the high suicide rates were kept secret and not reported to international organisations such as the WHO, as this did not fit with the image of a functioning socialism. With reunification after 1990, suicide rates in the former GDR fell dramatically, and in recent years, they have levelled off with decreasing rates in the West. Given the socioeconomic crisis years after reunification and the differences between East and West that still persist today, it cannot be assumed that the psychosocial burden on people in the former GDR has also fallen significantly. This means that suicides are also subject to completely different influences than primarily psychopathological characteristics. The reduction in suicide rates in East Germany is likely not due to a dramatic improvement in the mental health of the people living there.

On a completely different level, the pathologising view of suicidality is also experienced as an epistemic injustice in the discourse on disabilities. The concept of epistemic injustice, which is explained in more detail elsewhere and which has recently been increasingly discussed in psychiatry [42], describes the situation in which any other perspectives of the persons affected are not taken into account and are not heard in the scientific, political or legal realm. Analogous to racism, this discourse describes discrimination by non-disabled people (*ableism*) and healthy people (*sanism*) but also by people who are not suicidal [43]. Many people with suicidal experiences reject a pathologising view of this phenomenon as suicidism.

Finally, for the sake of completeness, it should also be mentioned that MAID is highly controversial in the disability movement. There are repeated fears that MAID is used as a means of pressurising people with disabilities to end their life because it places a burden on the family and causes costs. Empirically, however, this fear has little basis. Although there are no relevant studies related to psychosocial problems, data related to physical illness suggest that MAID is sought primarily by people with high social status and against a background of pronounced individuality and a lack of religious commitment [44, 45]. These studies suggest that social pressure does not appear to play a significant role.

2.5 Conclusion: The Decision-Making Dilemma of (Social) Psychiatry

How much room for manoeuvring do we give people who we diagnose as "severely mentally ill"? And is it justified to treat people with "severe mental illness" differently from people with physical illnesses, who may also have problems making illness-related decisions?

These questions lead psychiatry, but above all social psychiatry and mental health nursing, into a dilemma. On the one hand, people with severe psychosocial problems should be able to make decisions about their own affairs as independently and autonomously as possible. On the other hand, it is assumed that "mental disorder" can lead to decisions that may not be in the person's best interests. This is aggravated by the fact that political and legal positions, as well as associations of those affected, categorise decisions against a person's will as a violation of human rights according to the UN CRPD. Essentially, the question is what is considered pathological and to what extent "illness" or "disorder" can be used to legitimise interference with human rights.

The fact that this is not unproblematic is repeatedly emphasised in the relevant literature. It is not necessary to return to the positions of Thomas Szasz from the 1960s. The British psychiatrist George Szmukler recently noted the legitimisation problems of coercion in psychiatry on various occasions and suggested already in 2006 that these problems could be solved by legal means. His solution is that a common law (*fusion law*) is needed that does not discriminate between mental and non-mental illnesses but only takes mental capacity into account [46, 47]. Ultimately, however, his argument—which, in my view, is entirely understandable—has not been able to prevail, especially in psychiatry. The following chapter addresses in detail the reasons cited in psychiatry for legitimising measures against a person's will.

References

1. United Nations. UN convention on the rights of persons with disabilities. 2006. Available from: https://www.un.org/development/desa/disabilities/convention-on-the-rights-of-persons-with-disabilities/convention-on-the-rights-of-persons-with-disabilities-2.html.
2. Yakusheva O, van den Broek-Altenburg E, Brekke G, Atherly A. Lives saved and lost in the first six month of the US COVID-19 pandemic: a retrospective cost-benefit analysis. PLoS One. 2022;17(1):e0261759.
3. Ryan CJ, Bartels J. Involuntary hospitalization. In: Bloch S, Green SA, editors. Psychiatric ethics. 5th ed. Oxford: Oxford UP; 2021. p. 279–99.
4. Beauchamp TL, Childress JF. Principles of biomedical ethics. 8th ed. Oxford: Oxford UP; 2019.
5. Snellgrove BJ, Steinert T. Einwilligungsfähigkeit vor dem Hintergrund der UN-Behindertenrechtskonvention. Forens Psychiatr Psychol Kriminologie. 2017;11(3):234–43.
6. UN General Assembly. Report of the special rapporteur on torture and other cruel, inhuman or degrading treatment or punishment, Juan E Méndez. 2013. Contract No.: A/HRC/22/53.
7. UN General Assembly. Report of the Special Rapporteur on the right of everyone to the enjoyment of the highest attainable standard of physical and mental health. 2017. Contract No.: A/HRC/35/21.
8. WHO. Guidance on community mental health services: promoting person-centred and rights-based approaches. Geneva: World Health Organisation; 2021.
9. Galbert I, Azab AN, Kaplan Z, Nusbaum L. Staff attitudes and perceptions towards the use of coercive measures in psychiatric patients. Int J Ment Health Nurs. 2023;32(1):106–16.
10. Funk M, Bold ND. WHO'S QualityRights initiative: transforming services and promoting rights in mental health. Health Hum Rights. 2020;22(1):69–75.
11. Shakespeare T. The social model of disability. In: Davis LJ, editor. The disability studies reader. 2. London: Routledge; 2006. p. 197–204.
12. Reynolds JM. Theories of disability. In: Reynolds JM, Wieseler C, editors. The disability bioethics reader. New York: Routledge; 2022. p. 30–8.
13. Fitzpatrick JJ. Moral and ethical issues in mental health. Arch Psychiatr Nurs. 2016;30(6):647.
14. Barros S, Rodrigues J, Alves TC, Almeida AB. Nursing and the rights of people in the field of mental health. SciELO Brasil. 2021;75:e75suppl301.
15. Szasz TS. The myth of mental illness: foundations of a theory of personal conduct. New York: Harper; 1974.

16. Szasz TS. Open doors or civil rights for mental patients? J Individ Psychol. 1962;18(2):168–71.
17. Zinkler M, von Peter S. End coercion in mental health services—toward a system based on support only. Laws. 2019;8(3):19.
18. Gahr M, Spitzer M. Probleme einer psychiatrischen Versorgung ohne Zwang: Krankenhaus oder Gefängnis? Recht und Psychiatrie. 2020;38:135–7.
19. Brieger P, Menzel S. Psychiatrie ohne Ordnungsfunktion? – Kontra. Psychiatr Prax. 2020;47:297–8.
20. Die ST, der Psychiatrie D. Recht und. Psychiatrie. 2021;39:28–34.
21. Bundesverband Psychiatrie-Erfahrener, Bundesarbeitsgemeinschaft Psychiatrie-Erfahrener. Nicht in unserem Namen! Zur Kritik am Konzept einer freiwilligen Psychiatrie aus Betroffenenperspektive. Recht und Psychiatrie. 2021;39:35–8.
22. Szmukler G. "Capacity", "best interests", "will and preferences" and the UN convention on the rights of persons with disabilities. World Psychiatry. 2019;18(1):34–41.
23. Scholten M, Gather J. Adverse consequences of article 12 of the UN convention on the rights of persons with disabilities for persons with mental disabilities and an alternative way forward. J Med Ethics. 2018;44(4):226–33.
24. Appelbaum PS. Protecting the rights of persons with disabilities: an international convention and its problems. Psychiatr Serv. 2016;67(4):366–8.
25. Richter D. Assistierter Suizid/assistierte Selbsttötung für Menschen mit schweren psychischen Störungen – Pro. Psychiatr Prax. 2016;43(8):411–2.
26. Richter D. Unerträgliches Leiden und autonome Entscheidung: Warum Menschen mit psychischen Erkrankungen das Recht auf Sterbehilfe nicht verwehrt werden darf. In: Böhning A, editor. Assistierter Suizid für psychisch Erkrankte: Herausforderung für Psychiatrie und Psychotherapie. Bern: Hogrefe; 2021. p. 37–61.
27. AAS. "Suicide" is not the same as "Physician Aid in Dying": American Association of Suicidology. 2017. Available from: http://www.suicidology.org/Portals/14/docs/Press%20 Release/AAS%20PAD%20Statement%20Approved%2010.30.17%20ed%2010-30-17.pdf.
28. Gather J, Vollmann J. Suizidprävention und ärztlich assistierte Selbsttötung. Ein unauflösbarer ethischer Widerspruch für Psychiater? Nervenheilkunde. 2015;34:430–4.
29. Schmiedebach HP, Priebe S. Social psychiatry in Germany in the twentieth century: ideas and models. Med Hist. 2004;48(4):449–72.
30. Finzen A. Die neue Euthanasie in Belgien—Wie steht es um die psychisch Kranken? Psychiatr Prax. 2015;42:411–2.
31. Barbagli M. Farewell to the world: a history of Suicide. London: Polity Press; 2015.
32. Krumm S. Assistierter Suizid/assistierte Selbsttötung für Menschen mit schweren psychischen Störungen – Kontra. Psychiatr Prax. 2016;43(8):412–3.
33. Appelbaum PS. Should mental disorders be a basis for physician-assisted death? Psychiatr Serv. 2017;68(4):315–7.
34. Ducor P, Kiefer B. Grundsatz der Autonomie: ein letztes Sakrament? Schweizerische Ärztezeitung. 2018;99:910–2.
35. Morgan S, Andrews N. Positive risk-taking: from rhetoric to reality. J Ment Health Train Educ Pract. 2016;11(2):122–32.
36. Stefan S. Rational Suicide, Irrational Laws. Examining current approaches to Suicide in policy and law. New York: Oxford University Press; 2016.
37. Hjelmeland H, Dieserud G, Dyregrov K, Knizek BL, Leenaars AA. Psychological autopsy studies as diagnostic tools: are they methodologically flawed? Death Stud. 2012;36(7):605–26.
38. Franklin JC, Ribeiro JD, Fox KR, Bentley KH, Kleiman EM, Huang X, et al. Risk factors for suicidal thoughts and behaviors: a meta-analysis of 50 years of research. Psychol Bull. 2017;143(2):187–232.
39. Economou M, Madianos M, Theleritis C, Peppou LE, Stefanis CN. Increased suicidality amid economic crisis in Greece. Lancet. 2011;378(9801):1459.
40. Lopez Bernal JA, Gasparrini A, Artundo CM, McKee M. The effect of the late 2000s financial crisis on suicides in Spain: an interrupted time-series analysis. Eur J Pub Health. 2013;23(5):732–6.

References

41. von den Driesch E. Unter Verschluss: Eine Geschichte des Suizids in der DDR 1952–1990. Frankfurt M./New York: Campus; 2021.
42. Crichton P, Carel H, Kidd IJ. Epistemic injustice in psychiatry. British J Psychiatry Bullet. 2017;41(2):65–70.
43. Baril A. Suicidism: a new theoretical framework to conceptualize suicide from an anti-oppressive perspective. Disability Stud Quarterly 2020;40(3).
44. Battin MP, van der Heide A, Ganzini L, van der Wal G, Onwuteaka-Philipsen BD. Legal physician-assisted dying in Oregon and The Netherlands: evidence concerning the impact on patients in "vulnerable" groups. J Med Ethics. 2007;33(10):591–7.
45. Steck N, Junker C, Zwahlen M, for the Swiss National Cohort. Increase in assisted suicide in Switzerland: did the socioeconomic predictors change? Results from the Swiss National Cohort. BMJ Open. 2018;8(4):e020992.
46. Dawson J, Szmukler G. Fusion of mental health and incapacity legislation. Br J Psychiatry. 2006;188(6):504–9.
47. Szmukler G. Men in white coats: treatment under coercion. Oxford: Oxford University Press; 2018 01 Dec 2017.

The Legitimisation of Psychiatric Measures Against a Person's Will

3

3.1 Introduction

The treatment of people who were regarded as crazy, inappropriate or possessed probably involved certain forms of coercion in all phases of humanity. These people were excluded from social relationships, and they were locked up in various forms, just as strangers were regarded as barbarians and were fought against under certain circumstances. Historically, the aspect of involuntariness in dealing with people who displayed such "inadequate" behaviour can be seen as a constant. However, coercion has been legitimised in different ways over the last few centuries, which is linked to the development of psychiatric care, scientific ideas and social change in general.

Human rights have also been dealt with differently in different phases of the history of mental health care. As will be described in detail later in the book, two major phases can be recognised to date. The first phase lasted from the beginning of psychiatry as a science and as a medical discipline until well into the second half of the twentieth century. During this phase, which was largely characterised by institutions such as hospitals and asylums, human rights were largely disregarded. The institution-centred phase was followed by the "person-centred phase" from around the 1970s/1980s. Although human rights were now taken into account, the restriction of rights was justified on medical and ethical grounds.

3.2 Coercion in Psychiatric Care: The Institution-Centred Phase

Physical coercion and other measures against a person's will are therefore not only part of the present but also part of the past of psychiatry. The ancient Greek poet Aristophanes wrote that "madmen" were pelted with stones and Plato's "Laws" (section 934c7) contained a passage for dealing with "madness", which suggested that such people should be kept away from the public by their own family and that offences should be punished with fines [1]. Dealing with "madness" without coercion has never truly existed, at least in Europe, as can be surmised from these indications. The philosopher Michel Foucault characterised the institutionalised beginning of psychiatry in the seventeenth century as the "great confinement" [2]. Later historical research confirmed the aspect of confinement in psychiatry but shifted it to the end of the eighteenth century and the beginning of the nineteenth century and established a link with the Enlightenment. "(T)he history of psychiatry began as a history of custodial asylum, institutions to confine raging individuals who were dangerous to themselves and a nuisance to others" ([3]: 7). In custodial asylums, the idea of protection takes precedence over treatment. Even then, however, according to the historian Edward Shorter, the idea behind the "great confinement" was that placement in asylums against one's will could have a curative effect.

In addition to the history of psychiatry, the history of law is also highly important here. In the transition to the early modern period, the idea of a benevolent state that was allowed to make decisions about its subjects in certain situations prevailed in absolutist states. In the Anglo–Saxon legal tradition, this principle from Roman law was referred to as *parens patriae* [4]. The respective ruler was identical to the state and, according to this legal doctrine, also acted as a parent. As the terminology suggests, the *parens patriae* doctrine was predominantly applied in legal matters concerning the welfare of children. However, the principle of the benevolent state was also applied to people who were considered "mentally ill" [5]. In the United States, for example, it was regarded as a legal principle until well into the 1970s [6]. Although the principle was not referred to as such on the European continent, it was handled in a similar way under the concept of state "care" [7]. Involuntary placements are still called "welfare placements" (*fürsorgerische Unterbringungen*) in Switzerland today.

However, in nineteenth-century England, the nuisance to other people mentioned by Edward Shorter was possibly one of the main factors behind the establishment of *madhouses*, as they were known in the British Isles at the time. These were mainly privately funded institutions where wealthy families could house relatives who appeared to display unconventional behaviour and were therefore seen as a problem for the family's reputation. This unconventional behaviour was not only associated with what is now classified as mental illness but also involved socially offensive behaviour such as a liaison with a person from a lower social class or politically unpopular statements.

A prominent case in today's historical literature but also in the medical literature of the time, is known as the *Lanchester Case*. One of the best-known medical journals of the time, the *British Medical Journal*, reported that Edith Lanchester was institutionalised by a doctor at the instigation of her father and brothers [8]. The reasons given by the doctor for the compulsory measure were as follows: Miss Lanchester had started an "illicit relationship" with a man who was clearly below her social status and whom she did not intend to marry. She had also always been eccentric and had recently started to espouse socialist ideas. She was admitted to the asylum because she wanted to commit "social suicide" and was diagnosed with

3.2 Coercion in Psychiatric Care: The Institution-Centred Phase

"monomania" on the subject of marriage. Both the family doctor who was called in later and the medical specialists in the institution confirmed the hospitalisation, which was eventually rejected by the *Lunacy Commission*.

Other people were less fortunate. Here is an example that symbolises the fate of hundreds of thousands of people whose names have been forgotten: the writer Elsa Asenjieff was involuntarily admitted on the basis of the diagnosis "troublemaker delusion" (*Querulantenwahn*) in Leipzig, Germany, in the 1920s. She died in 1941 after several decades in hospitals and asylums. Medical-historical research has identified social background as a decisive factor in her tragic life story in Saxon psychiatry: "...as a single woman whose behaviour did not conform to social and gender norms and who had no family support, she already lived increasingly in poverty and isolation in the war-damaged young Weimar Republic" ([9]: 91).

This mixture of medical and social criteria for hospitalisation, which was generally involuntary, was applied in many countries until well into the second half of the twentieth century. At the end of the 1950s, an American psychiatrist described the traditional indications as follows:

> (1) behaviour which endangers the patient's life and (2) behaviour which the patient's environment will no longer tolerate. These classic indications for hospitalisation characteristics in common—both usually arise out of emergency situations, both are manifestations of severe degrees of mental illness. In either case, the patient does not seek hospitalisation himself—others seek it for him. And in either case the prescription for hospitalisation is usually made by the family, friends, judges, police—and of particular interest historically—rarely by a psychiatrist. The psychiatrist seldom disagrees with the lay prescription because the severity of the patient's illness and his need for hospital care are usually obvious. ([10]: 207)

Psychiatric institutions or asylums were established in almost all European countries during the nineteenth century. Those who were admitted often had to spend many years there. The conditions in most institutions are inhumane and socially and hygienically catastrophic. A few years after the end of the institution-centred phase, two German psychiatrists described this phase as a "...scandalous practice of asylums for the mentally ill and mentally handicapped in prison-like, oversised detention facilities that inevitably produced hospitalisation defects, whose equipment was mostly unworthy and whose staffing just allowed for supervision but no treatment..." ([11]: 588).

The historian Edward Shorter quotes a psychiatrist who worked at the Maudsley Hospital in London in the 1930s as saying, "Life was not quite so pleasant for the patients. Confined to locked wards with an enclosed garden for exercise, patients whose stormy illness had blown itself out, leaving only residual symptoms, would remain year after year, unoccupied, deprived of incentive or responsibility of self-determination, getting more and more fixed in the straitjacket of an unchanging daily routine" ([3]: 65f).

Most "inmates", as they were known at the time, had no rights with regard to therapy. They were, as the sociologist and historian Andrew Scull wrote, "...deprived of their status as moral actors, and presumed by virtue of their mental state to lack the capacity to make informed choice for themselves, patients were mostly unable to resist those who controlled their very existence…" ([12]: 308). Thus, sometimes brutal physical interventions were carried out against the will of those affected, from insulin shocks to surgical interventions in the brain (e.g. lobotomies) to electroconvulsive therapy, which were only carried out later under anaesthesia. The lack of rights was also one of the prerequisites for the murder of thousands of people with mental, cognitive and physical disabilities during National Socialism in Germany.

The associated ideas about people with mental health problems also dominated in former Eastern Germany. In 1979, Ehring Lange, one of the country's leading psychiatrists at the time, succinctly summarised the perceptions that still had to be overcome in the 1960s. A critical approach was needed:

> with the view that schizophrenic illnesses inevitably and irreversibly lead to a defect and that their core group should not be given special intensive treatment, with the view that a binding prognosis can be inferred from a cross-sectionally recorded symptomatology—which then predetermines the value or lack of value of therapy and rehabilitation, with the view that work therapy is a means of filling unused daytime for chronic institutionalised patients, but is superfluous for acutely ill patients in clinical treatment, with the view that the mentally ill person is fundamentally unpredictable, dangerous to himself and to the community owing to the inherent laws of the illness and therefore in principle requires closed accommodation and segregation from society. [13]

Thus, from today's perspective, abstruse judgements were not limited to the former GDR. "Mentally ill" people almost always act under pathological influences; therefore, there was no "inner freedom", and restrictions on movement were unproblematic, according to a medical opinion on the introduction of mental health laws in West Germany in the 1950s ([14]: 24). As part of the introduction of a legal framework for hospitalisation, there was also a discussion between legal and psychiatric experts about the involvement of courts in hospitalisation proceedings. On the medical side, there were fears of a restriction of medical therapeutic sovereignty and a strain on the therapeutic relationship ([14]: 24).

Many institutions in Eastern and Western Europe, which saw themselves as hospitals over the course of time, also took part in drug trials in which most patients were probably only asked for verbal consent at best; informal coercion can usually also be assumed in these cases. Until the 1960s, it was not common practice in all medical research to ask affected patients for consent [15]. Historical researchers in Switzerland documented these procedures for many psychiatric hospitals until well into the 1970s. These experiments with unauthorised medication resulted in numerous deaths, most of which were not documented or declared to relatives. The fact that negligent handling of consents also occurred among medical staff has become known in the context of the LSD trials at the Burghölzli University Hospital in Zurich. In 1947, staff were unknowingly given the substance in coffee [16]; in the case of patients on whom the "fantastic drug", as it was called at the time, was also tried, the corresponding article noted that they or their relatives had been asked for consent [17].

In general, medication was almost exclusively used as a treatment. Until the 1990s, for example, pronounced high-dose neuroleptic therapy was used [18], which was associated with considerable health problems for many patients. Symptoms were primarily suppressed, as this high-dose therapy already implies. Psychodynamic and later biomedical disease models dominated therapeutic reasoning. Surveillance and exclusion took priority over reintegration; there was no real rehabilitation. At best, those affected were transferred to other institutions, such as care homes and sheltered workshops. Physical needs were satisfied to some extent but slightly more than that. In professional training and research, people with "mental illnesses" were predominantly objects.

It was only from the 1950s in the United States and from the 1960s in Europe that conditions changed, albeit very slowly, as a report on a reform project in a state hospital in the United States from 1968 makes clear. It is also interesting to see how staff and the people locked up there treated each other: "Walls were painted, pictures and calendars had been introduced; and patients were given measures of dormitory and bathroom privacy. However, there was little concomitant change in the psychological architecture of the wards. Patients continued to fear staff, while staff continued to fear patients; patients retreated from the staff, who as often retreated from them. The staff felt hopeless about the patients, the patients felt hopeless about the staff" ([19]: 591f).

The legitimisation of coercion in this institution-centred phase was based on two intertwined lines of argument, which were, however, criticised even in legal circles from at least the 1960s onwards owing to their vague criteria and very flexible interpretations [20]. On the one hand, reference was made to the maintenance of public order. Particularly at the beginning of the phase from the end of the eighteenth century onwards, little emphasis was placed on the "state of mind"; public order was far more important. This then changed with the development of psychiatry as a medical discipline. In addition to the assumption that "mentally ill" people were "dangerous" and the resulting need for institutionalisation, a further justification was provided that is abstruse from today's perspective but still applies in certain variations to the present day: "mentally ill" people are not truly free due to their illness, so the deprivation of liberty through institutionalisation cannot be seen as such [14]. It is therefore hardly surprising that the persons affected by institutionalisation were generally not granted any rights. They were usually unable to refuse a doctor's order, were not given any information about the results of medical examinations and often did not know what medication they had to take [21].

3.3 From the Institution-Centred Phase to the Person-Centred Phase

"Negotiating instead of treating" (*Verhandeln statt Behandeln*) was the German-language motto of reform psychiatry, which at the same time described the core of care that was later referred to as person-centred support. The slogan was coined by the reform psychiatrist Asmus Finzen in the early 1990s, who wanted to clarify how social and community psychiatry differed from the institutional psychiatry of the time. As Finzen later wrote, it was the tangible "often experienced paternalism conducted by doctors" that motivated both service users and relatives to reject the traditional care system, which was sometimes associated with considerable coercion and human rights violations [22].

However, the 'person-centred approach' was not new in the 1990s when psychiatry discovered it. The basic idea came from one of the central figures in the history of psychotherapy, Carl Rogers, and was formulated back in the 1950s. According to Rogers, person-centredness, which is also known as client-centredness, has three essential characteristics of a therapeutic relationship [23]. The first is authenticity. This means, for example, dispensing with a professional façade and creating a congruent situation in which nobody pretends. The second characteristic is the creation of an accepting attitude that is non-judgemental and can therefore bring about change on the part of the client. Third, it is about empathic understanding, which is achieved through active listening, for example.

The concept of "patient-centred medicine" also dates back to the 1950s and 1960s and was propagated by the psychoanalyst Michael Balint as a contrast to "disease-centred medicine" [24]. According to this idea, the person to be treated should no longer be seen as just a person with a broken bone but as a "unique human being" who should receive an *overall diagnosis* and be treated accordingly.

Patient-centred medicine later became the core quality criterion for good medical care as a whole. In its 2001 report on quality deficiencies in healthcare, the US Institute of Medicine declared patient-centeredness to be one of the main objectives, along with other characteristics such as equity, safety, speed, effectiveness and efficiency [25]. According to the report, patient-centredness, in turn, has the following characteristics: (1) respect for patients' values and preferences, (2) coordination and integration of care, (3) information, communication and education, (4) physical well-being, (5) emotional support and (6) involvement of family and friends.

Over time, the aforementioned characteristics of patient- or person-centredness have increasingly been translated into skills that healthcare professionals such as doctors, nurses or therapists should learn as part of their training. Numerous studies have been conducted in this context, which have shown, on the one hand, that the skills can certainly be taught and applied by professionals but, on the other hand, that the effects on healthcare users cannot be measured so clearly, as seen in a large review from the Cochrane Initiative [26].

Another development that was already present in Balint's "patient-centred medicine" is the conceptual focus on the "person" and no longer on the "patient". This was intended to express that the person to be treated should be considered "holistically" and should not be reduced to the status of a patient. Person-centred care, according to one of the central theoretical contributions, is the "antithesis to reductionism" ([27]: 249). Methodologically, this involves two important elements: first, the story that the sick person has to tell and, second, *shared decision-making*. The latter has become increasingly central to person-centred care in recent years. The idea is that professionals and the person concerned, as well as other stakeholders such as relatives, should decide together for the benefit of all which treatment methods should be used.

However, what exactly was the difference between the community psychiatry of the reform years and the former institutional psychiatry? The Austrian sociologist Rudolf Forster summarised the reform efforts in the mid-1990s and described the project as follows [28]: Instead of a purely organic concept of illness, a multifactorial model was used that also contained psychosocial components. The aim was social integration instead of hospitalisation. Instead of medical dominance, a multiprofessional team was to advise on treatment. The legal basis should no longer be predominantly coercion but rather voluntariness. Instead of paternalistic directives on treatment, it was a partnership-based consultation that allowed the patients to decide—in other words, person-centredness.

Rudolf Forster came to a sobering conclusion at the end of his analysis. "The gap between claim and announcement on the one hand and the results and effects on the other is strikingly large in many reform projects" ([28]: 249). The reason for this, according to Forster, was quite clear: "Psychiatry has become above all a relatively *conventional medical discipline*" ([28]: 249; emphasis in original). Although psychiatry had changed in various respects and brought about many changes, medical dominance had not been fundamentally broken but had been consolidated by the fact that psychiatry had become increasingly similar to conventional medicine.

The integration of psychiatry into general medicine was not an accident of the reforms; it was the declared intention. In addition to the equalisation of the physically and mentally ill (as it was called at the time), the establishment of psychiatric wards in general hospitals in various countries, such as Italy and Germany, symbolised this integration. The aim was to change the special status and stigmatisation of psychiatric treatment through normalisation in medicine. However, psychiatry, and thus also social psychiatry, also aimed to normalise medicine conceptually, which meant, for example, a clear preference for pharmacotherapy over talk therapy [29]. It also meant a diagnostic model that described "mental illnesses" as part of general illnesses, for example, in the International Classification of Diseases (ICD), developed by the World Health Organisation. The ICD is used almost worldwide—with the exception of the United States—and mental disorders make up a central chapter.

Overall, it was an endeavour to treat less, i.e. to know and decide paternalistically what is good for the user, and to negotiate more, i.e. to attempt to arrive at a joint approach and make decisions "on an equal footing". The core of the endeavours, for example, in Germany, was "... the consistent orientation towards the individual support needs of the mentally ill person" ([30]: 8).

In principle, the concepts in both German-speaking and English-speaking countries were relatively unanimous. Person-centredness primarily meant finding out from service users what help they needed and meeting these needs as part of a coordinated help system involving community-based services. Other concepts from the early days of the person-centred approach envisaged a *Person-centred Integrative Diagnosis* (PID) for this purpose [31]. The PID was to cover the following aspects: positive and negative health aspects, which were to be assessed within the context of the person's life, social functions, protective factors, quality of life and information on dignity, values and motivations. However, all of this should be done within the framework of conventional classification systems such as the ICD. With reference to medical classification systems and treatment, it was made clear that person-centredness was still to be seen in a medical-psychiatric context.

In the 2010s, the concept of person-centredness underwent a change. With the recovery approach, the service user's perspective was generally incorporated more strongly into care. However, it is still unclear whether the combination of person-centredness and recovery would actually mean a fundamental change or whether recovery could be seamlessly integrated into person-centredness. There is still no consensus among experts on this topic. For example, it is argued that person-centredness should serve to support service users in the sense of recovery to lead a meaningful life [32]. Others see person-centredness together with recovery but also with the human rights approach as conceptual innovators in psychiatric care [33]. Third parties, in turn, see person-centredness as a culturally enriched, relationship- and recovery-oriented approach [34].

Other perspectives emphasise important differences. The recovery approach, which is already considered quasi-mainstream today, was notably not developed by clinicians but by those affected and those using it as a perspective that can run counter to medical understanding [35]. This is particularly the case when "illness" is no longer the central focus but rather the goal of leading a meaningful life despite or because of the illness, which does not necessarily mean adhering to psychiatric treatment methods and pharmacotherapy in particular. Recovery also favours support methods that are not considered evidence-based even in social psychiatry, such as the Open Dialogue method. Despite all the convergences with the person-centred approach, recovery is an approach that aims to achieve changes that are "consumer-driven" ([35]: 108). Overall, considerable ambivalence can be observed in current psychiatric care in this context. On the one hand, evidence-based care is upheld, while on the other hand, recovery and other concepts are propagated, at least programmatically.

3.4 The Legitimisation of Coercion in the Person-Centred Phase

One of the ambiguities of the concept of person-centredness is that it can go hand in hand with both recovery orientation and the perspective that healthcare professionals know what is good for the user. It is therefore not surprising that in the relevant literature, person- or patient-centredness is seen as a concept that should help to ensure that medication is taken consistently (e.g. in the adherence approach) [36]. It is just another step in a dubious direction when even coercive measures are discussed as potentially person-centred [37]. The fact that this abandons the idea of "equal footing" and shared decision-making on difficult issues in the context of treatment and care does not seem to matter.

Although a certain inconsistency or even abstruseness must be perceived here, it should be noted that this does not necessarily contradict conventional medical or psychiatric ethics. Person-centredness—as just described—also has a supposedly objectifiable side, and in conventional medical ethics, decisions are generally not made from the perspective of the person concerned but from an external perspective "for the good of the person concerned". This is also understandable insofar as many of the ethical situations to be discussed in acute medicine are based on the assumption that the persons concerned are unconscious and would consent to the measures. In legal terms, this is conceptualised as "natural will" [38].

This is somewhat different in psychiatric settings, as the people concerned are generally not unconscious. Historically, the views of the people responsible were certainly similar. Until the end of the last century, it was hardly questioned whether coercion could not be for the benefit of the person, especially as there was virtually no empirical research on this question in addition to the widespread paternalistic views. This was not to change until the mid-1990s, when ethical and professional discussions became much more important [39]. Over time, however, the conditions under which it could be ethically legitimised to treat people psychiatrically against their will were increasingly discussed. Is it sufficient to establish a medical need, or must the illness be associated with a risk to oneself, and what about risks to other people? Furthermore, what type of therapy may be used? Is electroconvulsive therapy also permitted against the patient's will, as was common practice for decades in the second half of the last century? All these issues, which were previously practised more or less unquestionably, have now been ethically and empirically analysed [40].

Furthermore, many countries have developed ethical and practical guidelines for dealing with suicidal behaviour and risk behaviour to others in psychiatric settings. There have even been attempts to harmonise this within a European framework [41].

In addition to professional and ethical aspects, legal considerations naturally play a central role in the legitimisation of coercion in psychiatric care. Both national and international courts and legal conventions have been increasingly concerned with this issue since the 1970s. According to a survey on the ethical and legal aspects of compulsory admission in 40 European countries, psychiatric coercion is currently legitimised by the combination of the presence of a "mental illness" and the risk to one's own health or the health of others [42]. The need for treatment as determined by medical professionals and significantly impaired judgement alone can also be used as justification in individual countries [43]. Furthermore, it is generally recognised that the measure should be a therapeutically effective intervention, that it should be used as a *last resort* and that it should be the *least restrictive alternative*. Overall, it is assumed that the measure is in the best interests of the person concerned.

The German Ethics Council has addressed this issue precisely in a comprehensive paper [44]. The document not only covers psychiatric issues in a narrower sense but also addresses other issues, such as how to regard age-related restrictions or involuntary measures in children and adolescents. The Ethics Council considers many of the measures used in psychiatry and other areas of healthcare to be ethically problematic but rejects a general renunciation of coercion in "professional care relationships", as one member of the Ethics Council explained: "In the view of the Ethics Council, coercive measures can be justified only if the person expresses wishes and needs for actions or the refusal of actions that threaten to seriously harm him or her but is not capable of making freely responsible decisions. A general rejection of all forms of coercive measures would lead to many vulnerable people being left to their fate. This is out of the question for the German Ethics Council" ([45]: 177).

Interestingly, the Ethics Council's opinion is that it only analyses coercion against the background of potential or actual harm to the individual. Dangers to other people were expressly not considered, although it is unclear for what reasons. One conceivable justification would be that medical intervention is not necessarily required to avert danger to other persons but that this would be possible in the context of police or judicial activities. However, no information was provided as to whether this justification applies, and it is therefore speculation.

In this context, the German Ethics Council is moving within the general framework of the ethical justification of coercion in psychiatry, as a systematic analysis of the arguments commonly used internationally has recently shown [46]. The ethical argumentation in favour of coercive measures in certain circumstances provides for the following aspects to be taken into account: autonomy and integrity are threatened by coercion but can also be restored by such a measure. The same applies to human dignity. Coercion can be used for the benefit of the person concerned (benevolence) and serves to avoid harm (non-maleficence). Coercion can also be fair insofar as individual and social interests are weighed. It can ultimately serve the safety of others as well as oneself and thus also be for the good of the greater whole.

In practice, these arguments also play a role. In general, in areas where coercion is used in psychiatry, the necessity and ultimately positive outcome of such measures are assumed. In addition, it is often argued that measures taken against a person's will also have therapeutic effects, such as promoting "insight into the illness" and compliance with treatment in general, as well as promoting the recovery process [47]. In addition, coercion serves to restore social order. However, in practice, such measures may jeopardise the therapeutic relationship [48, 49]. These negative consequences, which are also reflected in care settings, testify to ambivalence in dealing with coercive measures. Nevertheless, in practice, the arguments of necessity and the ultimate benefit for a person's well-being prevail [50].

The research literature on this topic draws attention to considerable social change that has also been reflected in care practice. Both in general psychiatric care and in forensic practice in particular, there has been a certain shift in many Western countries from primarily therapeutic aspects to safety aspects as well as risk assessment and risk avoidance [51, 52]. In this respect, it is hardly surprising that these aspects still play a strong role in the legitimisation of coercion in psychiatry today.

If one disregards the numerous country-specific characteristics in dealing with psychiatric coercion [42], the following schematic sequence emerges for the legitimisation of coercion in psychiatric contexts (Fig. 3.1).

The existence of a "mental disorder" with perceived impaired mental capacity or competence, combined with harm that has already occurred or a suspected risk to oneself or other persons, therefore justifies a coercive measure if it is used as a last resort and as the least restrictive measure possible. The overall measure is—so the assumption—in the interest and for the benefit of the person affected by the coercive

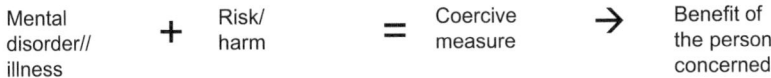

Fig. 3.1 Justification scheme for psychiatric coercive measures

measure, who would approve of the measure on the assumption of mental recovery or in hindsight. It is also assumed that the coercive measure is intended to restore the autonomy of the person concerned, which is considered to be significantly impaired by the mental disorder. This all presupposes that the therapy associated with coercion is effective and produces the desired results.

3.5 Conclusion: The Legitimisation of Coercion in Psychiatry: The Clinical-Ethical-Legal Stalemate

The legitimisation of coercion in psychiatry has changed considerably over the last few centuries, as the previous explanations have made clear. Whereas previously, the focus was on segregation and supposed dangerousness, this became much more medicalised and psychologised over the course of the twentieth century. Increasing emphasis has been placed on individual characteristics and backgrounds. However, this has not led to the abandonment of measures against the will of the person, as one might have assumed if the individuality of the person was better understood.

Medicalisation and psychologisation may have had the exact opposite effect. By focusing on the individual person, it may have been possible to better describe the risks that the person could pose. The same applies to the ethical discussion in general, which has manoeuvred itself into a dead end. The same ethical arguments, such as human dignity and the welfare of the person, can be used to argue both in favour of abolishing coercion and in favour of retaining it. Even clinical arguments can be made in favour of both the retention and abolition of coercion. If one side can legitimately argue that mental health problems can impair judgement, the other side can just as legitimately point out that the paternalistic treatment associated with coercion does not lead to the person's mental health and recovery. On a political and legal level, this situation has already been described as the Geneva impasse [53]. This refers to the fact that within the United Nations and the World Health Organisation (WHO), there are both conventions that legitimise coercion and those that attempt to abolish measures against a person's will. This means that even at the level of human rights, both sides are equipped with good arguments [54].

In this respect, ethical, legal, human rights and even clinical arguments do not truly help in the end. For an empirically orientated scientist such as me, part of the discussion is difficult to understand anyway, as the relevant empirical studies are often ignored. This will now be made up for. The question of whether coercion in psychiatry can be legitimised thus becomes an empirical question. It remains to be seen what studies and data are available to answer the question of whether coercion is actually for the benefit of the person concerned, for example. These empirical questions will be answered in the following chapter.

References

1. Thumiger C. Ancient Greek and roman traditions. In: Eghigian G, editor. The Routledge history of madness and mental health. London: Routledge; 2017. p. 42–61.
2. Foucault M. Folie et Déraison: Histoire de la folie à l'âge classique. Paris: Plon; 1961.
3. Shorter E. A history of psychiatry: from the era of the asylum to the age of Prozac. New York: Wiley; 1997.
4. Custer LB. The origins of the doctrine of Parens Patriae. Emory Law J. 1978;27:195–208.
5. Wesson M. Substituted judgment: the Parens Patriae justification for involuntary treatment of the mentally ill. J Psychiatry Law. 1980;8:147–65.
6. Zander TK. Civil commitment in Wisconsin: the impact of Lessard v Schmidt. Wis Law Rev. 1976;1976:503–62.
7. Müller M. Individuelle Selbstbestimmung und staatliche Fürsorge. Zeitschrift für Schweizerisches Recht. 2012;131:63–86.
8. BMJ. The Lanchester case. Br Med J. 1895:1127–8.
9. Kommol P, Steinberg H. Die Krankengeschichte Elsa Asenijeffs im Kontext des sächsischen psychiatrischen Anstalts- und Versorgungssystems der 1920er-Jahre bis 1941. Nervenarzt. 2022;93(1):86–92.
10. Hall BH. Prescribing hospitalization. Bull Menn Clin. 1958;22(6):207–13.
11. Thom A, Wulff E. Vergleichende Betrachtungen: Gemeinsamkeiten, Divergenzen und erkennbare Perspektiven struktureller Wandlungen der psychiatrischen Versorgungssysteme. In: Thom A, Wulff E, editors. Psychiatrie im Wandel: Erfahrungen und Perspektiven in Ost und West. Köln: Psychiatrie-Verlag; 1990. p. 587–602.
12. Scull A. Madness in civilization: a cultural history of insanity from the bible to Freud, from the madhouse to modern medicine. Princeton University Press: Princeton; 2015.
13. Lange E. Die Rodewischer Thesen 1963 – Vermächtnis und Verpflichtung, Bekenntnis und Verwirklichung. Psychiatr Neurol Med Psychol. 1979;31(7):385–92.
14. Bruns G. Ordnungsmacht Psychiatrie? Psychiatrische Zwangseinweisung als soziale Kontrolle. Opladen: Westdeutscher Verlag; 1993.
15. Miller FG. Clinical research before informed consent. Kennedy Inst Ethics J. 2014;24(2):141–57.
16. Rey C. Nach dem Zweiten Weltkrieg wird in Zürich Ärzten zu Forschungszwecken LSD heimlich in den Morgenkaffee gekippt. Neue Zürcher Zeitung. 2022 30.12.2022.
17. Stoll WA. Lysergsaure-diathylamid, ein Phantastikum aus der Mutterkorngruppe. Schweizer Archiv fur Neurologie und Psychiatrie. 1947;60(1–2):279–323.
18. Abrahamson D. High-dose antipsychotic medication. Br J Psychiatry. 1994;165(2):269.
19. Hirschowitz RG. Changing human behavior in the state hospital organization. Psychiatry Q. 1969;43(1):591–611.
20. Livermore JM, Malmquist CP, Meehl PE. On the justifications for civil commitment. Univ Pa Law Rev. 1968;117:75–96.
21. Tolchin G, Steinfeld G, Suchotliff L. The mental patient and civil rights: some moral, legal, and ethical considerations. Prof Psychol. 1970;1(3):212–6.
22. Finzen A. Über Behandlung verhandeln. Wege zu einer vertrauensvollen therapeutischen Beziehung 2010. Available from: http://www.finzen.de/pdf-dateien/behandlung_verhandeln.pdf
23. Rogers CR. The foundations of the person-centered approach. Education. 1979;100(2):98–107.
24. Balint E. The possibilities of patient-centered medicine. J R Coll Gen Pract. 1969;17(82):269.

References

25. Institute of Medicine Committee on Quality of Health Care in America. Crossing the quality chasm: a new health system for the 21st century. Washington: National Academies Press (US); 2001.
26. Dwamena F, Holmes-Rovner M, Gaulden CM, Jorgenson S, Sadigh G, Sikorskii A, et al. Interventions for providers to promote a patient-centred approach in clinical consultations. Cochrane Database Syst Rev. 2012;12:CD003267.
27. Ekman I, Swedberg K, Taft C, Lindseth A, Norberg A, Brink E, et al. Person-centered care – ready for prime time. Eur J Cardiovasc Nurs. 2011;10(4):248–51.
28. Forster R. Psychiatriereformen zwischen Medikalisierung und Gemeindeorientierung – Eine kritische Bilanz. Opladen: Westdeutscher Verlag; 1997.
29. Prosser A, Helfer B, Leucht S. Biological v. psychosocial treatments: a myth about pharmacotherapy v. psychotherapy. Br J Psychiatry. 2016;208(4):309–11.
30. Aktion Psychisch Kranke. Abschlussbericht des Projekts Implementation des personenzentrierten Ansatzes in der psychiatrischen Versorgung. Bonn: Aktion Psychisch Kranke; 2002.
31. Mezzich JE, Salloum IM. Towards innovative international classification and diagnostic systems: ICD-11 and person-centered integrative diagnosis. Acta Psychiatr Scand. 2007;116(1):1–5.
32. Martinelli A, Ruggeri M. An overview of mental health recovery-oriented practices: potentiality, challenges, prejudices, and misunderstandings. J Psychopathol. 2020;26:147–54.
33. Rosen A, Gill NS, Salvador-Carulla L. The future of community psychiatry and community mental health services. Curr Opin Psychiatry. 2020;33(4):375–90.
34. Gabrielsson S, Sävenstedt S, Zingmark K. Person-centred care: clarifying the concept in the context of inpatient psychiatry. Scand J Caring Sci. 2015;29(3):555–62.
35. Schmolke M, Amering M, Svettini A. Recovery, empowerment, and person centeredness. In: Mezzich JE, editor. Person centered psychiatry. Springer; 2016. p. 97–111.
36. Pyne JM, Fischer EP, Gilmore L, McSweeney JC, Stewart KE, Mittal D, et al. Development of a patient-centered antipsychotic medication adherence intervention. Health Edu Behav. 2014;41(3):315–24.
37. Rudnick A. Commentary: can seclusion and restraint be person-centered? Isr J Psychiatry Relat Sci. 2013;50(1):11–2.
38. Nossek A, Gather J, Vollmann J. Natürlicher Wille, Zwang und Anerkennung – Medizinethische Überlegungen zum Umgang mit nicht selbstbestimmungsfähigen Patienten in der Psychiatrie. Ethik Med. 2018;30(2):107–22.
39. Lidz CW. Coercion in psychiatric care: what have we learned from research? J Am Acad Psychiatry Law. 1998;26(4):631–7.
40. Tannsjo T. The convention on human rights and biomedicine and the use of coercion in psychiatry. J Med Ethics. 2004;30(5):430–4.
41. Kallert TW, Jurjanz L, Schnall K, Glöckner M, Gerdjikov I, Raboch J, et al. Eine Empfehlung zur Durchführungspraxis von Fixierungen im Rahmen der stationären psychiatrischen Akutbehandlung. Psychiatr Prax. 2007;34(Suppl 2):S233–40.
42. Wasserman D, Apter G, Baeken C, Bailey S, Balazs J, Bec C, et al. Compulsory admissions of patients with mental disorders: state of the art on ethical and legislative aspects in 40 European countries. Eur Psychiatry. 2020;63(1):e82.
43. Bartlett P. A mental disorder of a kind or degree warranting confinement: examining justifications for psychiatric detention. Int J Hum Rights. 2012;16(6):831–44.
44. German Ethics Council. Benevolent Coercion – Tensions between Welfare and Autonomy in Professional Caring Relationships. Berlin; 2018.
45. Graumann S. Pro: Hilfe durch Zwang? Professionelle Sorgebeziehungen im Spannungsfeld von Wohl und Selbstbestimmung. Eine Verteidigung der Stellungnahme des Deutschen Ethikrats. Ethik Med. 2019;31(2):175–9.
46. Chieze M, Clavien C, Kaiser S, Hurst S. Coercive measures in psychiatry: a review of ethical arguments. Front Psych. 2021;12:790886.

47. Paradis-Gagné E, Pariseau-Legault P, Goulet MH, Jacob JD, Lessard-Deschênes C. Coercion in psychiatric and mental health nursing: a conceptual analysis. Int J Ment Health Nurs. 2021;30(3):590–609.
48. Gerace A, Muir-Cochrane E. Perceptions of nurses working with psychiatric consumers regarding the elimination of seclusion and restraint in psychiatric inpatient settings and emergency departments: an Australian survey. Int J Ment Health Nurs. 2019;28(1):209–25.
49. Theodoridou A, Schlatter F, Ajdacic V, Rössler W, Jäger M. Therapeutic relationship in the context of perceived coercion in a psychiatric population. Psychiatry Res. 2012;200(2):939–44.
50. Morandi S, Silva B, Mendez Rubio M, Bonsack C, Golay P. Mental health professionals' feelings and attitudes towards coercion. Int J Law Psychiatry. 2021;74:101665.
51. Doedens P, Vermeulen J, Boyette LL, Latour C, de Haan L. Influence of nursing staff attitudes and characteristics on the use of coercive measures in acute mental health services-a systematic review. J Psychiatr Ment Health Nurs. 2020;27(4):446–59.
52. Oosterhuis H, Loughnan A. Madness and crime: historical perspectives on forensic psychiatry. Int J Law Psychiatry. 2014;37(1):1–16.
53. Martin W, Gurbai S. Surveying the Geneva impasse: coercive care and human rights. Int J Law Psychiatry. 2019;64:117–28.
54. Richter D. Coercion in psychiatry: the human rights challenge. In: Hallett N, Whittington R, Richter D, Eneje E, editors. Coercion and violence in mental health settings: causes, consequences, management. Cham: Springer Nature Switzerland; 2024. p. 173–90.

Psychiatric Coercion: Ethical Conditions and Empirical Data

4.1 Introduction

Modern society knows various forms of coercion. These range from the threat of fines, such as those related to compulsory seat belt use in cars or a smoking ban on aeroplanes, to the deployment of a special police task force to put an end to a hostage situation. Psychiatric coercion is a variant of general societal coercion. Since psychiatric coercion formally takes place in the context of medical care, it requires special legitimisation, as described in the previous chapter. One of the most important ethical and legal arguments for the justification of coercion in medicine in general and in psychiatry in particular is that the measure must ultimately be for the benefit of the person concerned. The person concerned should, according to the aforementioned criterion of the German Ethics Council, realise in retrospect that the measure was justified and that they benefited from it insofar as the absence of the measure would have led to harm to health. This also implies the effectiveness of the entire treatment. In addition, the measure must be used as a last resort when all others have been exhausted, and it must be the least restrictive possible. Finally, it is assumed that the measure restores the person's autonomy. However, is this truly the case? What does empirical research say about ethical conditions? The following conditions for the use of psychiatric coercion are therefore considered below:

1. Coercion is for the benefit of the person concerned.
2. The least possible restriction is used as a last resort.
3. Psychiatric therapies are effective.
4. The coercive measure restores the autonomy of the person concerned.

Another fundamental condition is the presence of a mental illness. As this topic is very complex and multi-faceted, it is addressed in detail in the next chapter.

© The Author(s), under exclusive license to Springer Nature
Switzerland AG 2025
D. Richter, *Human Rights in Psychiatry*,
https://doi.org/10.1007/978-3-031-98635-2_4

4.2 Condition 1: Is Coercion for the Benefit of the Person Concerned?

Do people affected by coercive measures agree afterwards with what has happened? Does the stay or even the treatment against their will help them in terms of their health? And what about people who are unable to enter the primary labour market or get their own flat because they are denied this on the grounds of a mental disorder and supposedly for their own good? Do they ultimately benefit from this?

Before these questions can be answered in detail, it is first necessary to consider the perspective from which a person's welfare should be viewed. From an ethical and legal perspective, as has already been stated on various occasions, it is the perspective of the person concerned. However, in practice but also in research, this is not always the case. A systematic review of coercion in the context of diagnosed eating disorders, for example, concluded that the measures are justified, as people affected by coercion would improve their body mass index just as much as those treated voluntarily [1]. This view is also paradigmatic for forensic psychiatry. There, among other things, the risk of criminal recidivism is seen as a main parameter of treatment outcomes [2]. Although this is presumably also the view of some of the people affected, there are considerable doubts as to whether this is the case for the majority. The clinical view, which does not necessarily take into account the perspective of the people affected, continues to dominate in practice but also, to some extent, in law.

However, let us stick to the clinical perspective first. What are the effects of involuntary measures? Various reviews have analysed the short-term effects of chemical restraints. They unanimously conclude that these measures work as intended and are able to actually calm affected—usually aggressive or agitated—people [3–5]. The side-effect profile and safety of the measures are also rated as positive [6].

But what about the longer-term effects? Interestingly, the relevant review literature is much less positive. With regard to the clinical effects of involuntary hospitalisation, a recently published scoping review concluded: "The clinical outcomes of IPA (Involuntary Psychiatric Admission; DR) are a highly conflicting and debated topic" ([7]: 291). On the one hand, minor psychopathological symptoms are emphasised, while on the other hand, depressive, post-traumatic and suicidal reactions are highlighted. A somewhat older review on restraint came to the conclusion that "... restraint is still widely used in psychiatry wards (3.8–20%) even though its efficacy has not been demonstrated..." ([8]: 19). A lack of effectiveness is also attested to for coercive outpatient measures, which are known as community treatment orders (CTOs). These are particularly ineffective with respect to readmissions to inpatient treatment and other parameters of the utilisation of psychiatric services [9, 10].

The reviews just cited have a crucial methodological problem in that they cannot control that the same characteristics of the people in the intervention group and in the control group are actually present in the conditions to be compared. Strictly speaking, this is only possible in the case of randomised clinical trials (RCTs). However, random allocation to a group that is subject to coercion and one for which

4.2 Condition 1: Is Coercion for the Benefit of the Person Concerned?

this is not the case is impossible, not least for ethical reasons. One way out of this problem is the so-called emulation study, in which an RCT is copied to a certain extent by means of an observational study [11].

In this way, it is possible to come relatively close to the "gold-standard" RCT without performing randomisation. This emulation procedure was applied to two datasets, one from a hospital and one from a national dataset from Switzerland. The primary outcome indicator was the clinical assessment by practitioners on the Health of the Nation Outcome Scale (HoNOS). Both in the hospital [12] and in the national database [13], patients who had to undergo coercive measures had significantly worse HoNOS scores. In other words, even from an exclusively professional clinical perspective, patients with a coercive measure deteriorate significantly.

Now to the perspective of those affected by coercion. Numerous empirical studies have focused primarily on the effects of direct coercion, and there are now various systematic literature reviews on this issue. Among these systematic reviews, one review has explicitly focused on ethical problems and their consequences. As already mentioned in connection with the German Ethics Council, the welfare of the person concerned is regarded by the ethical literature as "...the most important justification for coercion" ([14]: 99). For example, antipsychotic medication against the person's will is considered justified because it is assumed to be better than no medication at all. However, as this review concludes, "although beneficence may be the justification, this may not ultimately be the case" ([14]: 100). This ethically motivated study also emphasises the extent to which coercion adversely affects the relationship between professionals and those affected and how much mistrust arises on the part of those affected.

A qualitative meta-synthesis has summarised the experiences of people who were initially hospitalised against their will and then had to undergo further coercive measures such as seclusion/isolation or restraint. The analysis yields the following conclusions, which are quoted extensively owing to their relevance:

> Patients in several studies believed that their involuntary admission had kept them safe at a time when they could not recognise the severity of their illness, but negative experiences were commonly described. (...) Additionally, this review found physical interventions, such as restraint and seclusion, were experienced particularly negatively by many patients and played an important role in the negative experiences reported in the majority of studies. This review also highlights the lasting impact of detention with a number of patients across studies reporting feelings of shame and marginalisation, particularly patients in forensic settings who had committed an offence as well. ([15]: 7)

Another systematic review analysed the consequences of restraint and seclusion/isolation for the people affected [16]. As this review is, in my opinion, the most comprehensive analysis, the summary from the discussion of the article is also quoted here at greater length:

> The identified literature strongly suggests that seclusion and restraint have deleterious physical or psychological consequences. The incidence of PTSD after seclusion or restraint ranges from 25% to 47%, which is not negligible, especially in patients with past traumatic events. The main diagnoses associated with the use of seclusion or restraint in the selected

articles are schizophrenic, schizoaffective, or bipolar, currently manic disorders. Subjective perception has high interindividual variability and can be positive, with feelings of safety, help, clinical improvement, or evaluation as necessary. However, seclusion and restraint are mostly associated with negative emotions, particularly feelings of punishment and distress. Conclusions on protective or therapeutic effects of seclusion and restraint are more difficult to draw. Our results provide little evidence for these outcomes, but further research is clearly necessary. ([16]: 13; citations not reproduced here)

A systematic review of qualitative studies focused exclusively on the effects of seclusion. This review concludes the following: "Thematic synthesis of the data revealed emotionally powerful themes which suggest that seclusion is an exceptionally challenging experience for psychiatric inpatients. (…) The process of it is frightening for patients and leaves them in a vulnerable state with inadequate resources available to help them to cope with the distress" ([17]: 281).

Yet another review examined the details of the experiences of people affected by coercive measures [18]. This work comes to a similar conclusion to the study just cited. The majority of experiences associated with coercive measures are negative, regardless of the type of measure. The following experiences are described in detail: Anxiety and post-traumatic stress; powerlessness, neglect, mistrust and loneliness; punishment, abuse and pain; anger, rage and bitterness; depression, grief; humiliation and shame; and loss of freedom and coercion. However, positive experiences such as help and support, necessity, reassurance, time to reflect, safety, control and prevention of violence were also reported in a smaller number of the original studies. In this overall context, it should also be borne in mind that physical restraint not only has psychological consequences but also—albeit rarely—leads to physical harm and even death [19, 20]. Deaths are usually caused by cardiac arrest, pulmonary embolism or thromboembolism.

The predominantly negative experiences apply not only to acute psychiatry but also, in particular, to forensic institutions. The summarised results of a review are also quoted here in full:

> In the available literature, restrictive practices have been associated with harmful consequences for users, including feelings of anger, aggression and anxiety as well as experiencing trauma, disorientation and experiencing neglect and abuse. (…) (R)estrictive practices can become part of a 'vicious circle' in which the psychological instability and stress they create lead to more risk-taking behaviour, which in turn leads to restrictive practices. ([21]: 80)

This corresponds with another review of studies from the forensic setting. There, the experience of many of those affected is summarised as a culture of "repression" [22]. Against this background, it is understandable that more contemporary concepts such as personal recovery find it relatively difficult to gain a foothold in forensic settings [23]. The prevailing rules and norms, the duration of the placement and, finally, the attitudes of the staff, which often tend towards a conventional ideology of punishment, obviously stand in the way of the development of an individual perspective of hope.

4.2 Condition 1: Is Coercion for the Benefit of the Person Concerned?

Other reviews of individual aspects of the experience of coercion are largely along the same lines as the work just cited [4, 24–29]. The majority of people affected do not experience psychiatric coercion as benevolent. However, there is apparently a minority of people affected by coercion who view this positively, and there are apparently certain situations in which people have experienced placement as a form of security.

These results are related to direct and ultimately physical coercion. However, according to a corresponding overview, even informal or "soft" coercion also leads to negative experiences. Furthermore, it is not surprising if the feeling of inferiority in the sense of fewer rights and less freedom of choice than other people arises [30].

In the introductory chapter, I referred to the problem of social coercion, which occurs when people are denied certain life prospects through administrative decisions, i.e. when people are not supported in entering the primary labour market or when people are denied living in their own home with reference to their mental health problems.

Unfortunately, there are no studies on the effects of these forms of coercion. This is probably because the withholding of life prospects has not yet been categorised as coercion. Nevertheless, statements can be made about the consequences of people with psychosocial problems not being employed in the primary labour market and the consequences of living in residential care or group settings.

The idea that people with psychosocial problems are not as resilient and have to adapt slowly to difficulties dates back to the early days of psychiatric rehabilitation. These ideas are referred to as the "stepladder principle" [31] or the "linear continuum" [32]. This is based on the expectation that people with psychosocial problems—as in other areas of medical rehabilitation—become increasingly burdened to recover. This means that they should move up from the workshop via a social or supplementary employment company into the general labour market. Alternatively, it means moving from a residential care setting via an assisted living community into one's own home.

However, unlike in many other medical fields, this step ladder principle does not work. As empirical studies have shown, only 10–15% of people actually achieve their goals via the step ladder [33, 34]. In contrast, the success rate for the principle of "supported inclusion", i.e. direct access to the labour market and one's own home, is significantly better [34–38]. For many people who are unable to gain a foothold in the primary labour market, this means that they have to live at or below the poverty line. This is the case for almost half of the people with severe psychosocial problems in Switzerland [39]. Social exclusion through poverty may even have increased in recent decades, as a Belgian study recently documented [40]. For people who cannot live in their own home, these "objective" disadvantages are not visible. However, the preference against a residential or shared flat setting is so pronounced that in a research project in which I was involved, we had to virtually discontinue the study because hardly anyone was willing to voluntarily live in such a setting for a longer period of time [36]. Surveys of people with pronounced psychosocial problems have shown that more than 80% of respondents opt for their own home [41]. To summarise, this means that the well-being of the person concerned is difficult to achieve in the case of social coercion. The disadvantages of social exclusion in terms of working and contravening the preference for housing are more than clear.

Is coercion associated with benefits for the people affected? The answer is both from the clinical perspective of professionals and from the perspective of those affected, predominantly no. Coercion is obviously only experienced as helpful by a minority of affected people. Evidence-based medicine is based on the view that a medical intervention is, on average, more successful than no intervention or an alternative treatment ("average treatment effect"). From this perspective, psychiatric coercion is not evidence-based, as the people affected—on average—do not benefit. Therefore, the discussion about psychiatric coercion should actually be over at this point. As the benefits cannot be proven, coercion in psychiatry should no longer be legitimised.

4.3 Condition 2: Is the Least Possible Restriction Used, and Is It Used as a Last Resort?

Coercive measures in psychiatry should be avoided wherever possible. If they are used, other options must have been considered and rejected. However, is this truly the case? To answer these questions, we can only partially draw on systematic reviews. It is first necessary to look at what resources are available as alternatives in psychiatric care.

Coercive measures usually arise either as a reaction to an escalating situation outside the inpatient setting or as a reaction to a—usually—aggressive conflict in the hospital. Let us first look at the situations in hospitals. In most psychiatric institutions in the Western world, measures have now been established in which staff can learn organisational and personal strategies to reduce coercive measures. These measures range from de-escalation training to improved and individualised therapy and care planning. Systematic reviews have shown that these measures tend to have a positive effect. An umbrella review summarising several meta-analyses revealed that employee training alone is able to minimise restraints [42]. However, if training alone is sufficient to achieve this effect, then this is an empirical indication that restraints are apparently not always used as a last resort, as more and better training is able to reduce coercion.

Further confirmation of this fact came from a large randomised implementation study of guidelines for reducing coercion in Germany. This showed a reduction in coercive measures in both the intervention group and the control group [43]. This circumstance, known in empirical research as the "Hawthorne effect", can be interpreted to mean that even in the control group, taking part in a study apparently had a positive impact on the use of coercion. In other words, there would have been room for less coercion even before the study.

However, coercion reduction initiatives often cannot achieve what was intended [44]. This also applies to the currently best-known programme *Safewards*. Safewards aims to reduce conflicts in inpatient facilities and thus indirectly reduce restrictions

4.3 Condition 2: Is the Least Possible Restriction Used, and Is It Used as a Last Resort?

and coercive measures. Two recently published reviews reported a tendency to reduce these measures, but this was not the case in all the studies included [45, 46]. This means that it is possible to use certain alternatives before interventions such as restraint or seclusion/isolation are used.

However, the question is how well this works in everyday practice. We know that studies are one thing; routine practice is another. So-called wash-out effects often occur. This means that the effect disappears over time after the intervention has been introduced, with a certain amount of effort and attention. Reviews [47] and individual studies [48, 49] suggest that there is indeed still considerable room for improvement here. Many of those affected primarily perceive the attempt to prevent formal coercive measures via medication and indirect coercion, such as threats of consequences. However, from the point of view of those affected, this is not particularly helpful. Instead, the focus is on dialogue and asking about current needs. In contrast, employees are generally convinced that they have used the last resort [50]. However, they do not see these means as exclusively related to the persons directly affected. In their opinion, coercive measures are also used to restore security and order in the respective department [51, 52].

Another way of applying fewer restrictions, which has not been used sufficiently to date, is to open closed wards. Closed ward doors are intended to prevent people from absconding from the ward or hospital and then possibly committing acts that are dangerous to themselves or others. However, it has been known for decades how much closed doors lead to aggressive conflicts in psychiatric wards [53]. There are no high-quality reviews on the subject of door openings, but both long-term retrospective observational studies [54] and prospective quasi-experimental studies [55] are available. These studies suggest that opening the door is not associated with an increased risk of suicide or other adverse events. A Norwegian study explicitly tested this non-inferiority with a corresponding study design and was able to impressively confirm the non-inferiority of open doors [56].

From the point of view of reducing coercion in hospitals, much would therefore be gained if the risk of hospitalisation could be reduced in advance. The intervention of choice is so-called "home treatment", which is described in German social law as "ward-equivalent treatment" and is known in British care as the "Crisis Resolution Team" [57]. Home treatment has been introduced in many countries, albeit with major differences and varying degrees of success [58]. Most home treatment programmes, such as those in Switzerland [59] and the Netherlands [60], succeed in reducing inpatient treatment days but not admissions. This is presumably due to the exclusion criteria for treatment in the home environment, which provide for inpatient admission if a certain risk threshold is exceeded.

In addition, however, home treatment programmes are not yet widespread outside the British Isles. In Switzerland, they only exist in a few locations, and even in Germany, where "ward-equivalent treatment" has been announced with great vigour, the number of cases is a single-digit percentage of all treatment cases [61].

In many cases, home treatment may also take place too late to prevent hospitalisation. The escalation may often already be too far advanced. A comprehensive study of the risk factors for involuntary admission in Switzerland, involving several thousand cases, revealed how relevant the factors of aggressiveness and on the part of those affected contribute to the risk of admission [62]. Various systematic reviews have shown the relevance of so-called advance directives in this context [63, 64]. These are measures that create trust that the support system will fulfil the wishes of the affected person, even in the context of a serious psychosocial crisis. According to the reviews cited, these measures are actually the only ones that contribute significantly to less coercion.

A residential support programme that takes place in advance could also help prevent crises from developing by building trust in the support system and providing support with everyday problems. Indeed, as reviews suggest, such programmes appear to do this [65, 66]. In our recent supported housing study in Zurich and Bern from 2020 to 2022, we explicitly examined this phenomenon and were able to clearly confirm a reduction [36]. In another study with a different sample, we were also able to show that residential coaching (as we call it in Bern) significantly reduced the risk of inpatient admission [67].

Ultimately, the aim is to extend the continuum of approaches to crisis intervention so that the appropriate response can be given to people seeking help and that they are not deterred by the threat of coercive measures when they are looking for support [68]. This also includes services such as peer respites [69] or crisis cafés [70], which can offer low-threshold counselling and support and dispense with immediate clinical measures, which might then automatically lead to psychiatric coercion.

To summarise, there are, in principle, measures available both in inpatient and outpatient settings, but they are not currently used consistently enough or across the board. Despite all the efforts on the part of professionals, it cannot be concluded that the principles of last resort and least possible restriction are actually followed in every case.

4.4 Condition 3: Is Psychiatric Treatment Effective?

Coercive measures in the psychiatric support system have the ultimate goal of contributing to the health of the people affected by the measures. It is therefore not about the defence against a risk or harm but about the therapeutic effectiveness of the entire treatment associated with the measure. However, how effective is psychiatric treatment? Admittedly, this is not the first time this question has been asked in connection with coercive measures. As early as 1987, Mary Durham and John La Fond addressed the following analytical questions in the context of the US legal system and the US federal government's efforts at the time to restrict the rights of people with mental health problems after years of deinstitutionalisation: "Does it in fact help the individuals whom the government is purportedly seeking to help? Is there any evidence to establish that it does? Is there evidence that such persons might in fact be harmed rather than helped?(...) [I]t is crucial that available empirical evidence be carefully scrutinized to see if the government can in fact carry its strong burden of demonstrating that it is able to accomplish the therapeutic purpose

4.4 Condition 3: Is Psychiatric Treatment Effective?

for which it seeks to take away the liberty of a vast number of Americans" ([71]: 309f). The answers the researchers gave were sobering. Instead of a therapeutic benefit, the findings at the time were more of a harm to people affected by coercion, for example, owing to the considerable side and long-term effects of the drugs.

However, what is the situation today and in view of the considerable changes in psychiatric therapy? A recently published umbrella review has provided an answer to this question [72]. In this type of review, a statistical methodology is applied to published systematic meta-analyses. The study therefore does not include individual studies, as in a normal meta-analysis but rather includes aggregated data from the reviews. Such umbrella reviews are particularly useful when many meta-analyses have already been published in a field of research such as psychiatric therapy research.

The aforementioned study included studies that covered 3700 randomised controlled studies with over 650,000 participants from noncoercive settings; the study therefore has considerable significance because of the number of studies included. The umbrella review then looked at how effective both pharmacological and psychotherapeutic interventions were in relation to standardised psychopathological scales. The decisive indicator is the standardised mean difference, which in turn corresponds to the effect size of an intervention (Cohen's d; see [73]). This indicates how large the measured differences between the intervention groups and the control groups were. The intervention groups received the drug or therapy that was tested, and the control groups received the placebo drug or usual care (TAU, *treatment as usual*).

The standardised mean difference, i.e. the overall effect size of the pharmacological interventions, was 0.34 for psychotherapy and 0.36 for pharmacotherapy. An effect size of 0.5 or more is usually considered to be moderately effective, and 0.8 or more is considered to be highly effective. This means that psychiatric therapy, whether pharmacotherapy or psychotherapy, is not even moderately effective. Only a minority of people who are treated actually benefit from the treatment.

The size of this minority in pharmacotherapy with antidepressants was recently calculated as part of a meta-analysis [74]. This analysis was based on data from the US *Food and Drug Administration* (FDA). The advantage of this database is that no publication bias is expected in the data to be analysed. In meta-analyses of only published studies, there is the phenomenon particularly in pharmacological research, when studies without success for the intervention are sometimes not published and therefore cannot be included in meta-studies. On the basis of FDA data on antidepressant monotherapy, an effect beyond the placebo effect was shown in only 15% of those treated. Not to be misunderstood: this is not nothing, and I would also try an antidepressant myself first in the event of a depressive development. However, I have serious doubts as to whether this rather small effect can be used as justification for an effective psychiatric intervention, which in turn can be used to justify a possible coercive measure.

In the context of coercive measures, it should also be noted that the study participants are exclusively volunteers, who can be assumed to have a certain motivation to be treated and to change. In the case of involuntary treatment, this motivation, if it exists at all, is significantly lower; therefore, an even lower level of effectiveness must be assumed here.

Another effect that leads to an overestimation of the reported effectiveness of psychopharmacological interventions is the empirical finding that participants in RCTs show better effectiveness than do those in so-called real-world studies [75]. The reason for this lies in the relatively strict inclusion criteria of RCT studies, which, among other things, mean that people with psychosocial problems who have multiple diagnoses (comorbidities) are generally excluded. The exclusion is intended to relate the measured effectiveness to the particular psychological problem and to avoid confounding factors.

Suicidality is the most common indication for coercive psychiatric measures, alongside risk and aggression to others. It is therefore worth examining the effectiveness of therapeutic interventions with respect to suicidality and completed suicides. A comprehensive meta-analysis with RCTs from 50 years with all possible interventions revealed an effect size that cannot even be interpreted as small (Hedge's $g = 0.17$) [76]. As with the effect size Cohen's d, from 0.2 onwards, we speak of a small effect, and from 0.5 onwards, we speak of a moderate effect. Two things were particularly interesting about this study in addition to the central result: first, no intervention was identified that was significantly more effective in the treatment of suicidality than others were, and, second, there was virtually no evidence about the effectiveness of acute psychiatric treatment, as is usually associated with compulsory hospitalisation due to suicidality.

Another meta-analysis focused on pharmacological and somatic interventions such as electroconvulsive therapy [77]. This analysis revealed significant effects on completed suicides only for lithium for people diagnosed with bipolar disorder and clozapine for people diagnosed with psychotic disorder. All other antipsychotics and electroconvulsive therapy showed no significant results. Yet another meta-analysis focused on pharmacological interventions. This showed a low effect size of 0.21 across all the medication classes [78]. However, researchers have emphasised the possible negative effects of certain medications, which can even increase the risk of suicide. A corresponding meta-analysis reported this for the selective serotonin reuptake inhibitor (SSRI) class of antidepressants [79].

For the sake of completeness, it should be emphasised that psychotherapeutic procedures also have only minor effects on suicidality, as a recent review has shown [80]. The same applies to brief aftercare contacts following discharge from inpatient treatment. These transitional interventions were able to influence suicidality to a small extent but did not affect the likelihood of completing suicide [81].

I already noted at the beginning of this chapter that criteria are applied in the context of compulsory admission and compulsory treatment, which are not necessarily relevant from the perspective of the person concerned. Corresponding meta-analyses from forensic settings report, among other things, positive developments in criminal recidivism. However, they also reported a comparatively high suicide mortality rate among people who were released from forensic treatment [82]. In line with the umbrella study described above, psychotherapeutic and pharmacotherapeutic reviews from forensic institutions have also emerged with only weak effects

[83] or had to concede that the original studies were not very meaningful [84]. A similar situation can be observed when reviews of psychotherapeutic and pharmacotherapeutic interventions for individuals diagnosed with disorders, such as dissociality or sexual offences, are examined. There is hardly any evidence of effective procedures for either [85–87].

In addition to forensic institutions, various individual studies have been conducted on the outcomes of involuntary treatment, but I was only able to identify two systematic reviews. One of these is not entirely new [88], and the other summarises only studies from Norway [89]. Both studies contain a large number of studies with heterogeneous outcome indicators, which, unfortunately, are not particularly informative for the research question.

The legal question cited at the beginning regarding the benefits of psychiatric therapy in the context of coercive measures must therefore continue to be answered as rather questionable. Against the background of the evidence referred to in condition 1, a benefit that is to be assessed as low must be set against an expected harm for the persons affected by coercion.

4.5 Condition 4: Can the Autonomy of the Persons Concerned Be Restored?

A central generalised assumption when deciding on coercive measures is the reduced autonomy of the person concerned. It is believed that "mental illness" impairs the ability to form self-determined and free will. The person's decisions against treatment are therefore overridden by the illness. Conversely, the treatment associated with the measure aims to restore autonomy, which is postulated accordingly in the legal literature [90, 91]. However, is this even possible? Is autonomy diminished by the illness, and can it be restored?

To answer these questions, we are only partially involved in empirical research. The problems of autonomy and free will are mainly discussed in philosophy. The problem for the question at hand here, however, is that these terms—as is often the case in philosophy—have very different meanings [92]. However, this applies not only to theoretical analyses but also to everyday life in psychiatric institutions. While from a medical perspective, a person's autonomy is impaired by the illness [93], affected persons are more likely to experience that their autonomy is reduced by coercive measures [94].

What is the significance of autonomy and free will in the context of psychiatry? Reduced culpability in connection with a psychosocial problem is an issue that is particularly familiar with legal proceedings. This issue, known as the *insanity defence*, is particularly relevant in criminal proceedings when defendants are not sentenced to the usual punishment but instead receive other forms of punishment owing to their mental state, such as therapy conditions or placement in a forensic setting. Ultimately, diminished culpability is used as a construct to avoid injustice and to protect people with pronounced psychosocial problems from a prison sentence [95].

From a human rights perspective, the distinction between people who have committed offences under the influence of a mental health problem and those for whom this was not the case is certainly problematic. There is even a view that sees this as discrimination and demands equal treatment [96]. In this respect, the question of whether actions are fundamentally autonomous and conditioned by free will or whether this is not the case is of fundamental importance.

In philosophy, certain perspectives involve autonomy and free will in a relevant context. Autonomous decisions are, according to one view, determined by free will [97]. However, as might be expected, this view is not uncontroversial [98]. A fundamental discussion revolves around the question of whether actions and decisions are biologically determined. Since every sequence in a cascade to an action is preceded by other steps, the debate centres on how much freedom can actually exist. In addition to this determinism/indeterminism debate, there is another debate about the extent to which a deterministic view does not enable free will. It is therefore about the compatibility of determinism and free will.

From a purely scientific point of view, indeterminism and the compatibility of determinism and free will are not fundamentally excluded [99], but they are hardly plausible. The biologist Robert Sapolsky once dryly remarked that free will is what biology has not yet discovered [100]. From an overall perspective, I do not necessarily adopt this perspective if I find it plausible. To summarise the question at hand, this means that from a philosophical perspective and from a neuroscientific perspective, it is at least unclear whether humans have something like autonomy and free will at all. In fact, in my personal opinion, there is a great deal to suggest that this is not the case. However, if it is at least unclear that people even have a form of autonomy that can be impaired by a mental disorder, then there are also very serious doubts as to whether psychiatric therapy can restore this autonomy through coercive measures.

Elsewhere, the previously cited biologist Robert Sapolsky expressed the hope "... that when it comes to dealing with humans whose behaviors are among our worst and most damaging, words like 'evil' and 'soul' will be as irrelevant as when considering a car with faulty brakes..." ([101]: 611). If the mechanics experts cannot find a source of the fault and the defect persists, we will not be talking about a "bad car" either, Sapolsky continues.

If I think this example through further, this means that just as the question of further use arises with cars, the question must be asked with people with dangerous tendencies as to how they can be dealt with in a humane way so that they pose as little danger as possible to their fellow human beings. I attempt to answer this question in Chap. 8. It should already have become clear here that a relatively deterministic view of the human psyche does not necessarily have to result in dehumanisation. According to Sapolsky, such a way of thinking "... is a hell of a lot more humane than demonizing and sermonizing them as sinners" ([101]: 612).

4.6 Conclusion: Ethical Assumptions and Empirical Data

The above remarks should clarify how much the ethical assumptions and justifications differ from the results of the relevant empirical research. Psychiatric coercion is predominantly not carried out for the benefit of the person concerned. Additionally, measures against the will are generally not used as a last resort and as the least possible restriction. There are usually more options than are implemented in the respective care systems. There is considerable doubt about the effectiveness of psychiatric therapies in general, especially in the context of involuntary settings. There are at least many doubts regarding the assumption that a person's autonomy can be restored by means of coercive measures. Another important prerequisite for the use of coercion in psychiatric settings, namely, the definition of a mental disorder, remains to be clarified. This is done in the following chapter.

References

1. Atti AR, Mastellari T, Valente S, Speciani M, Panariello F, De Ronchi D. Compulsory treatments in eating disorders: a systematic review and meta-analysis. Eat Weight Disord. 2021;26(4):1037–48.
2. Hachtel H, Vogel T, Huber CG. Mandated treatment and its impact on therapeutic process and outcome factors. Front Psych. 2019;10:10.
3. Muir-Cochrane E, Grimmer K, Gerace A, Bastiampillai T, Oster C. Safety and effectiveness of olanzapine and droperidol for chemical restraint for non-consenting adults: a systematic review and meta-analysis. Australas Emerg Care. 2021;24(2):96–111.
4. Muir-Cochrane E, Oster C. Chemical restraint: a qualitative synthesis review of adult service user and staff experiences in mental health settings. Nurs Health Sci. 2021;23(2):325–36.
5. Zun LS. Evidence-based review of pharmacotherapy for acute agitation. Part 1: onset of efficacy. J Emerg Med. 2018;54(3):364–74.
6. Zun LS. Evidence-based review of pharmacotherapy for acute agitation. Part 2: safety. J Emerg Med. 2018;54(4):522–32.
7. Iudici A, Girolimetto R, Bacioccola E, Faccio E, Turchi G. Implications of involuntary psychiatric admission: health, social, and clinical effects on patients. J Nerv Ment Dis. 2022;210(4):290–311.
8. Beghi M, Peroni F, Gabola P, Rossetti A, Cornaggia CM. Prevalence and risk factors for the use of restraint in psychiatry: a systematic review. Riv Psichiatr. 2013;48(1):10–22.
9. Kisely SR, Campbell LA, O'Reilly R. Compulsory community and involuntary outpatient treatment for people with severe mental disorders. Cochrane Database Syst Rev. 2017;3
10. Barnett P, Matthews H, Lloyd-Evans B, Mackay E, Pilling S, Johnson S. Compulsory community treatment to reduce readmission to hospital and increase engagement with community care in people with mental illness: a systematic review and meta-analysis. Lancet Psychiatry. 2018;5(12):1013–22.
11. Hernán MA, Robins JM. Using big data to emulate a target trial when a randomized trial is not available. Am J Epidemiol. 2016;183(8):758–64.
12. Baggio S, Kaiser S, Wullschleger A. Effect of seclusion on mental health status in hospitalized psychiatric populations: a trial emulation using observational data. Eval Health Prof. 2024;47(1):3–10.
13. Baggio S, Kaiser S, Huber CG, Wullschleger A. Effect of coercive measures on mental health status in adult psychiatric populations: a nationwide trial emulation. Epidemiol Psychiatr Sci. 2024;33:e35.

14. Hem MH, Gjerberg E, Husum TL, Pedersen R. Ethical challenges when using coercion in mental healthcare: a systematic literature review. Nurs Ethics. 2018;25(1):92–110.
15. Akther SF, Molyneaux E, Stuart R, Johnson S, Simpson A, Oram S. Patients' experiences of assessment and detention under mental health legislation: systematic review and qualitative meta-synthesis. Br J Psych Open. 2019;5(3):e37.
16. Chieze M, Hurst S, Kaiser S, Sentissi O. Effects of seclusion and restraint in adult psychiatry: a systematic review. Front Psych. 2019;10:491.
17. Askew L, Fisher P, Beazley P. What are adult psychiatric inpatients' experience of seclusion: a systematic review of qualitative studies. J Psychiatr Ment Health Nurs. 2019;26(7–8):274–85.
18. Aguilera-Serrano C, Guzman-Parra J, Garcia-Sanchez JA, Moreno-Küstner B, Mayoral-Cleries F. Variables associated with the subjective experience of coercive measures in psychiatric inpatients: a systematic review. Can J Psychiatr. 2018;63(2):129–44.
19. Kersting XAK, Hirsch S, Steinert T. Physical harm and death in the context of coercive measures in psychiatric patients: a systematic review. Front Psych. 2019;10:400.
20. Steinberg A. Prone restraint cardiac arrest: a comprehensive review of the scientific literature and an explanation of the physiology. Med Sci Law. 2021;61(3):215–26.
21. Lawrence D, Bagshaw R, Stubbings D, Watt A. Restrictive practices in adult secure mental health services: a scoping review. Int J Forensic Ment Health. 2022;21(1):68–88.
22. Tomlin J, Bartlett P, Völlm B. Experiences of restrictiveness in forensic psychiatric care: systematic review and concept analysis. Int J Law Psychiatry. 2018;57:31–41.
23. Bredenoort M, Roeg DPK, van Vugt MD. A shifting paradigm? A scoping review of the factors influencing recovery and rehabilitation in recent forensic research. Int J Law Psychiatry. 2022;83:101812.
24. Tingleff EB, Bradley SK, Gildberg FA, Munksgaard G, Hounsgaard L. "Treat me with respect". A systematic review and thematic analysis of psychiatric patients' reported perceptions of the situations associated with the process of coercion. J Psychiatr Ment Health Nurs. 2017;24(9–10):681–98.
25. Cusack P, Cusack FP, McAndrew S, McKeown M, Duxbury J. An integrative review exploring the physical and psychological harm inherent in using restraint in mental health inpatient settings. International Jorunal of Mental Health Nursing. 2018;27(3):1162–76.
26. Sugiura K, Pertega E, Holmberg C. Experiences of involuntary psychiatric admission decision-making: a systematic review and meta-synthesis of the perspectives of service users, informal carers, and professionals. Int J Law Psychiatry. 2020;73:101645.
27. Modini M, Burton A, Abbott MJ. Factors influencing inpatients perception of psychiatric hospitals: a meta-review of the literature. J Psychiatr Res. 2021;136:492–500.
28. Mellow A, Tickle A, Rennoldson M. Qualitative systematic literature review: the experience of being in seclusion for adults with mental health difficulties. Ment Health Rev J. 2017;22(1):1–15.
29. Lindgren B-M, Ringnér A, Molin J, Graneheim UH. Patients' experiences of isolation in psychiatric inpatient care: insights from a meta-ethnographic study. Int J Ment Health Nurs. 2019;28(1):7–21.
30. Allison R, Flemming K. Mental health patients' experiences of softer coercion and its effects on their interactions with practitioners: a qualitative evidence synthesis. J Adv Nurs. 2019;75(11):2274–84.
31. Richter D, Hertig R, Hoffmann H. Psychiatrische rehabilitation – von der Stufenleiter zur unterstützten Inklusion. Psychiatr Prax. 2016;43(8):444–9.
32. Ridgway P, Zipple AM. The paradigm shift in residential services: from the linear continuum to supported housing approaches. Psychosoc Rehabil J. 1990;13(4):11–31.
33. Killaspy H, Priebe S, McPherson P, Zenasni Z, Greenberg L, McCrone P, et al. Predictors of moving on from mental health supported accommodation in England: national cohort study. Br J Psychiatry. 2020;216(6):331–7.
34. Richter D, Hoffmann H. Effectiveness of supported employment in non-trial routine implementation: systematic review and meta-analysis. Soc Psychiatry Psychiatr Epidemiol. 2019;54(5):525–31.

References

35. Suijkerbuijk YB, Schaafsma FG, van Mechelen JC, Ojajarvi A, Corbiere M, Anema JR. Interventions for obtaining and maintaining employment in adults with severe mental illness, a network meta-analysis. Cochrane Database Syst Rev. 2017;9:CD011867.
36. Mötteli S, Adamus C, Deb T, Fröbel R, Siemerkus J, Richter D, et al. Independent supported housing for non-homeless people with serious mental illness: a pragmatic randomized controlled trial. Front Psych. 2021;12:798275.
37. Dehn LB, Beblo T, Richter D, Wienberg G, Kremer G, Steinhart I, et al. Effectiveness of supported housing versus residential care in severe mental illness: a multicenter, quasi-experimental study. Soc Psychiatry Psychiatr Epidemiol. 2022;57(5):927–37.
38. Adamus C, Mötteli S, Jäger M, Richter D. Independent supported housing for non-homeless individuals with severe mental illness: comparison of two effectiveness studies using a randomised controlled and an observational study design. Front Psych. 2022;13:1033328.
39. Richter D, Hoffmann H. Social exclusion of people with severe mental illness in Switzerland: results from the Swiss health survey. Epidemiol Psychiatr Sci. 2019;28(4):427–35.
40. Smith P, Nicaise P, Lorant V. Social integration of people with non-psychotic mental illness over the last 2 decades: the widening gap in the adult population in Belgium. Soc Psychiatry Psychiatr Epidemiol. 2022;33
41. Richter D, Hoffmann H. Preference for independent housing of persons with mental disorders: systematic review and meta-analysis. Admin Pol Ment Health. 2017;44(6):817–23.
42. Barbui C, Purgato M, Abdulmalik J, Caldas-de-Almeida JM, Eaton J, Gureje O, et al. Efficacy of interventions to reduce coercive treatment in mental health services: umbrella review of randomised evidence. Br J Psychiatry. 2021;218(4):185–95.
43. Steinert T, Baumgardt J, Bechdolf A, Bühling-Schindowski F, Cole C, Flammer E, et al. Implementation of guidelines on prevention of coercion and violence (PreVCo) in psychiatry: a multicentre randomised controlled trial. Lancet Regional Health Europe. 2023;35:100770.
44. Väkiparta L, Suominen T, Paavilainen E, Kylmä J. Using interventions to reduce seclusion and mechanical restraint use in adult psychiatric units: an integrative review. Scand J Caring Sci. 2019;33(4):765–78.
45. Finch K, Lawrence D, Williams MO, Thompson AR, Hartwright C. A systematic review of the effectiveness of Safewards: has enthusiasm exceeded evidence? Issues Ment Health Nurs. 2022;43(2):119–36.
46. Mullen A, Browne G, Hamilton B, Skinner S, Happell B. Safewards: an integrative review of the literature within inpatient and forensic mental health units. Int J Ment Health Nurs. 2022;31(5):1090–108.
47. Lincoln TM, Heumann K, Teichert M. Das letzte Mittel? Ein Überblick über die politische Diskussion und den Forschungsstand zum Einsatz medikamentöser Zwangsbehandlung in der Psychiatrie. Verhaltenstherapie. 2014;24(1):22–32.
48. Heumann K, Bock T, Lincoln TM. Bitte macht (irgend)was! Eine bundesweite Online-Befragung Psychiatrieerfahrener zum Einsatz milderer Maßnahmen zur Vermeidung von Zwangsmaßnahmen. Psychiatr Prax. 2017;44(2):85–92.
49. Heumann K, Stückle L, Jung A, Bock T, Mahlke C, Lincoln TM. Wählen wir die richtigen Mittel zur Zwangsvermeidung? Eine Befragung von psychiatrischen PatientInnen mit Zwangserfahrung zur potenziellen Nützlichkeit Milderer Mittel. Psychiatr Prax. 2021;48(6):301–8.
50. Riahi S, Thomson G, Duxbury J. A hermeneutic phenomenological exploration of 'last resort' in the use of restraint. Int J Ment Health Nurs. 2020;29(6):1218–29.
51. Paradis-Gagné E, Pariseau-Legault P, Goulet MH, Jacob JD, Lessard-Deschênes C. Coercion in psychiatric and mental health nursing: a conceptual analysis. Int J Ment Health Nurs. 2021;30(3):590–609.
52. Doedens P, Vermeulen J, Boyette LL, Latour C, de Haan L. Influence of nursing staff attitudes and characteristics on the use of coercive measures in acute mental health services-a systematic review. J Psychiatr Ment Health Nurs. 2020;27(4):446–59.
53. Nijman HLI, Allertz WFF, Merckelbach HLGJ, Ravelli DP. Aggressive behaviour on an acute psychiatric admissions ward. Eur J Psychiatry. 1997;11:106–14.

54. Huber CG, Schneeberger AR, Kowalinski E, Fröhlich D, von Felten S, Walter M, et al. Suicide risk and absconding in psychiatric hospitals with and without open door policies: a 15 year, observational study. Lancet Psychiatry. 2016;3(9):842–9.
55. Schreiber LK, Metzger FG, Flammer E, Rinke H, Fallgatter AJ, Steinert T. Open doors by fair means: a quasi-experimental controlled study on the effects of an open-door policy on acute psychiatric wards. BMC Health Serv Res. 2022;22(1):941.
56. Indregard A-MR, Nussle HM, Hagen M, Vandvik PO, Tesli M, Gather J, et al. Open-door policy versus treatment-as-usual in urban psychiatric inpatient wards: a pragmatic, randomised controlled, non-inferiority trial in Norway. Lancet Psychiatry. 2024;11(5):330–8.
57. Wheeler C, Lloyd-Evans B, Churchard A, Fitzgerald C, Fullarton K, Mosse L, et al. Implementation of the crisis resolution team model in adult mental health settings: a systematic review. BMC Psychiatry. 2015;15:74.
58. Holgersen KH, Pedersen SA, Brattland H, Hynnekleiv T. A scoping review of studies into crisis resolution teams in community mental health services. Nord J Psychiatry. 2022:1–10.
59. Stulz N, Wyder L, Maeck L, Hilpert M, Lerzer H, Zander E, et al. Home treatment for acute mental healthcare: randomised controlled trial. Br J Psychiatry. 2020;216(6):323–30.
60. Cornelis J, Barakat A, Blankers M, Peen J, Lommerse N, Eikelenboom M, et al. The effectiveness of intensive home treatment as a substitute for hospital admission in acute psychiatric crisis resolution in The Netherlands: a two-Centre Zelen double-consent randomised controlled trial. Lancet Psychiatry. 2022;9(8):625–35.
61. GKV-Spitzenverband VD, Krankenhausgesellschaft D. Gemeinsamer Bericht über die Auswirkungen der stationsäquivalenten psychiatrischen Behandlung im häuslichen Umfeld auf die Versorgung der Patientinnen und Patienten einschließlich der finanziellen Auswirkungen gemäß § 115d Absatz 4 SGB V. 2021.
62. Silva B, Gholam M, Golay P, Bonsack C, Morandi S. Predicting involuntary hospitalization in psychiatry: a machine learning investigation. Eur Psychiatry. 2021;64(1):e48.
63. de Jong MH, Kamperman AM, Oorschot M, Priebe S, Bramer W, van de Sande R, et al. Interventions to reduce compulsory psychiatric admissions: a systematic review and meta-analysis. JAMA Psychiatry. 2016;73(7):657–64.
64. Molyneaux E, Turner A, Candy B, Landau S, Johnson S, Lloyd-Evans B. Crisis-planning interventions for people with psychotic illness or bipolar disorder: systematic review and meta-analyses. Br J Psych Open. 2019;5(4):e53.
65. McPherson P, Krotofil J, Killaspy H. Mental health supported accommodation services: a systematic review of mental health and psychosocial outcomes. BMC Psychiatry. 2018;18(1):128.
66. Richter D, Hoffmann H. Independent housing and support for people with severe mental illness: systematic review. Acta Psychiatr Scand. 2017;136(3):269–79.
67. Adamus C, Zürcher SJ, Richter D. A mirror-image analysis of psychiatric hospitalisations among people with severe mental illness using independent supported housing. BMC Psychiatry. 2022;22(1):492.
68. Dangwung P, Golden K, Webb A, Fredrick M, Roberts DL. The UT health living room: expanding the psychiatric crisis continuum of care. Community Ment Health J. 2024;60(8):1589–95.
69. Oostermeijer S, Morgan A, Cheesmond N, Green R, Reavley N. The effects of Australia's first residential peer-support suicide prevention and recovery Centre (SPARC). Crisis. 2024;45(3):217–24.
70. Staples H, Cadorna G, Nyikavaranda P, Maconick L, Lloyd-Evans B, Johnson S. A qualitative investigation of crisis cafés in England: their role, implementation, and accessibility. BMC Health Serv Res. 2024;24(1):1319.
71. Durham ML, La Fond JQ. A search for the missing premise of involuntary therapeutic commitment: effective treatment of the mentally ill. Rutgers Law Review. 1987;40:303–68.
72. Leichsenring F, Steinert C, Rabung S, Ioannidis JPA. The efficacy of psychotherapies and pharmacotherapies for mental disorders in adults: an umbrella review and meta-analytic evaluation of recent meta-analyses. World Psychiatry. 2022;21(1):133–45.

73. Andrade C. Mean difference, standardized mean difference (SMD), and their use in meta-analysis: as simple as it gets. J Clin Psychiatry. 2020;81(5)
74. Stone MB, Yaseen ZS, Miller BJ, Richardville K, Kalaria SN, Kirsch I. Response to acute monotherapy for major depressive disorder in randomized, placebo controlled trials submitted to the US Food and Drug Administration: individual participant data analysis. Br Med J. 2022;378:e067606.
75. Efthimiou O, Taipale H, Radua J, Schneider-Thoma J, Pinzón-Espinosa J, Ortuño M, et al. Efficacy and effectiveness of antipsychotics in schizophrenia: network meta-analyses combining evidence from randomised controlled trials and real-world data. Lancet Psychiatry. 2024;11(2):102–11.
76. Fox KR, Huang X, Guzmán EM, Funsch KM, Cha CB, Ribeiro JD, et al. Interventions for suicide and self-injury: a meta-analysis of randomized controlled trials across nearly 50 years of research. Psychol Bull. 2020;146(12):1117–45.
77. Wilkinson ST, Trujillo Diaz D, Rupp ZW, Kidambi A, Ramirez KL, Flores JM, et al. Pharmacological and somatic treatment effects on suicide in adults: a systematic review and meta-analysis. Depress Anxiety. 2022;39(2):100–12.
78. Huang X, Harris LM, Funsch KM, Fox KR, Ribeiro JD. Efficacy of psychotropic medications on suicide and self-injury: a meta-analysis of randomized controlled trials. Transl Psychiatry. 2022;12(1):400.
79. Hengartner MP, Amendola S, Kaminski JA, Kindler S, Bschor T, Plöderl M. Suicide risk with selective serotonin reuptake inhibitors and other new-generation antidepressants in adults: a systematic review and meta-analysis of observational studies. J Epidemiol Community Health. 2021;75(6):523–30.
80. Teismann T, Gysin-Maillart A. Psychotherapie nach einem Suizidversuch – Evidenzlage und Bewertung. Bundesgesundheitsbl Gesundheitsforsch Gesundheitsschutz. 2022;65(1):40–6.
81. Tay JL, Li Z. Brief contact interventions to reduce suicide among discharged patients with mental health disorders—a meta-analysis of RCTs. Suicide Life Threat Behav. 2022;52(6):1074–95.
82. Fazel S, Fimińska Z, Cocks C, Coid J. Patient outcomes following discharge from secure psychiatric hospitals: systematic review and meta-analysis. Br J Psychiatry. 2016;208(1):17–25.
83. Ross J, Quayle E, Newman E, Tansey L. The impact of psychological therapies on violent behaviour in clinical and forensic settings: a systematic review. Aggress Violent Behav. 2013;18(6):761–73.
84. Howner K, Andiné P, Engberg G, Ekström EH, Lindström E, Nilsson M, et al. Pharmacological treatment in forensic psychiatry – a systematic review. Front Psych. 2020;10
85. Khalifa NR, Gibbon S, Völlm BA, Cheung N-Y, McCarthy L. Pharmacological interventions for antisocial personality disorder. Cochrane Database Syst Rev. 2020;9
86. Adshead G, McGauley G. Psychotherapy of psychopathic disorders. In: The Wiley International handbook on psychopathic disorders and the law; 2020. p. 835–63.
87. Hoberman HM. Forensic psychotherapy for sexual offenders: has its effectiveness yet been demonstrated? In: Phenix A, Hoberman HM, editors. Sexual offending: predisposing antecedents, assessments and management. New York: Springer New York; 2016. p. 605–66.
88. Katsakou C, Priebe S. Outcomes of involuntary hospital admission – a review. Acta Psychiatr Scand. 2006;114(4):232–41.
89. Wynn R. Involuntary admission in Norwegian adult psychiatric hospitals: a systematic review. Int J Ment Heal Syst. 2018;12(1):10.
90. Haydt N. The DSM-5 and criminal defense: when does a diagnosis make a difference? Utah law. Review. 2015:847–80.
91. Winick BJ. Ambiguities in the legal meaning and significance of mental illness. Psychol Public Policy Law. 1995;1(3):534–611.
92. Müller S, Walter H. Reviewing autonomy: implications of the neurosciences and the free will debate for the principle of respect for the patient's autonomy. Camb Q Healthc Ethics. 2010;19(2):205–17.

93. Radoilska LV. Personal autonomy, decisional capacity, and mental disorder. In: Radoilska L, editor. Autonomy and mental disorder. Oxford: Oxford University Press; 2012. p. ix–xli.
94. Bennion E. A right to remain psychotic-a new standard for involuntary treatment in light of current science. Loyola Los Angeles Law Rev. 2013;47:251–318.
95. Malatesti L, Jurjako M, Meynen G. The insanity defence without mental illness? Some considerations. Int J Law Psychiatry. 2020;71:101571.
96. Minkowitz T. Rethinking criminal responsibility from a critical disability perspective: the abolition of insanity/incapacity acquittals and unfitness to plead, and beyond. Griffith Law Rev. 2014;23(3):434–66.
97. Weissman D. Autonomy and free will. Metaphilosophy. 2018;49(5):609–45.
98. Pereboom D. Free will. Cambridge: Cambridge University Press; 2022.
99. Glannon W. Free will in light of neuroscience. In: Glannon W, editor. Free will and the brain: neuroscientific, philosophical, and legal perspectives. Cambridge: Cambridge University Press; 2015. p. 3–24.
100. Sapolsky RM. Neuroscience and the law. University St Thomas J Law Public Policy. 2021;15:138–61.
101. Sapolsky RM. Behave – the biology of humans at our best and worst. London: Bodley Head; 2017.

Mental Disorder: What Is It and How Valid Is the Definition?

5.1 Introduction

In the previous chapter, we looked at various criteria on the basis of empirical research results that are used to legitimise coercive measures. Now, it is a matter of a further and absolutely central criterion, which is listed in the "equation" in Fig. 3.1. The use of coercion in psychiatric care, as it exists today, requires the identification of a mental disorder or mental illness. If people are considered "too ill" in the psychiatric sense, then, in the opinion of many professionals, it is justified not only in psychiatry in general but also in social psychiatry and mental health nursing to restrict the autonomy of the persons concerned, which is actually held in high regard, and to use coercion under certain circumstances.

In other words, despite the inclination of professionals, who certainly understand the preferences of the people concerned, the latter often prevails when weighing up autonomy vs. the concept of illness. Logically, two main questions need to be answered positively to justify coercion in psychiatric care: [1] Is the definition of a mental illness/disorder valid enough? [2] Can a sufficient distinction be made between "mental health" and "mental illness"? In my view, the second question in particular is essential to be able to legitimise admitting people to psychiatric care against their will and, if necessary, treating them. I attempt to answer these questions below. The fact that this is an attempt already shows how difficult this terrain is that we are about to enter. The terrain lies somewhere between psychology, neuroscience, sociology and, above all, philosophy.

Three topics are considered in this context. The first is the question of what we know about the existence of the human psyche. Second is the distinction between mental illness on the one hand and what can be vaguely described as healthy or non-ill on the other. Third, we look at how mental illnesses or disorders are currently classified, for example, how they are differentiated from one another.

© The Author(s), under exclusive license to Springer Nature
Switzerland AG 2025
D. Richter, *Human Rights in Psychiatry*,
https://doi.org/10.1007/978-3-031-98635-2_5

5.2   Is There Even a Human Psyche?

First, the aspect of an illness or disorder should be left out. If we ask ourselves what a mental illness is, we should—again logically—ask whether there is a mental realm, psyche or human mind that can become ill, or what we know about the existence of the human psyche or mind. "A mental disorder is a condition of mind. It is mind-dependent. If no mind existed, no mental disorder could exist" ([1]: 12).

In our everyday lives, we probably consider this question to be completely meaningless; in our everyday understanding, we do not question whether there is a human psyche, soul or spirit. We all experience more or less pleasant emotional moments, and it is clear to all of us that we can perceive, think and draw conclusions, i.e. that we have cognitive characteristics that are also part of the human psyche. This is our everyday understanding, and when we work as professionals in psychiatry, psychotherapy or mental health nursing, it is usually also our clinical understanding. In addition—as will be analysed in more detail later—this does not have to be wrong. Interestingly, however, terms such as "psyche" and "soul" are at best cited only historically in more recent research literature. This is particularly the case when basic neuroscientific research is involved. There may be different opinions about basic neuroscientific research, but this kind of research is central to the current scientific understanding of the psyche and therefore also of mental illness. Even if you—like me—come from a social science background, you cannot ignore these findings [2].

In basic neuroscientific research and in associated philosophical research, the question of the existence of the psyche has, to a certain extent, already been shelved; the talk there is primarily "consciousness" (for philosophy, e.g [3].; for the neurosciences, [4]). Unlike psyche and soul, consciousness is regarded as a scientifically accessible topic that can be analysed empirically and theoretically. Instead of soul and psyche, scientists today tend to speak of mind and consciousness. Despite this semantic change from psyche to mind in the relevant research, the term "psyche" is still used in clinical and colloquial language. For this reason, I use the terms "psyche" and "mind" interchangeably and on an equal footing, unless other characteristics are mentioned.

With the shift towards a scientific approach to consciousness, one would think that the secrets of the brain and of thinking and feeling have been quickly decoded. This is certainly true for individual questions of detail. However, the central questions of consciousness, and above all, the problem of the emergence of consciousness as something subjective, seem to be no less solved today than in earlier times. This subjectivity is—if you like—the essence of consciousness. In one of the most quoted philosophical articles of the second half of the twentieth century, the American philosopher Thomas Nagel asked in the 1970s what it was like to be a bat. His answer: We do not know, and we will never be able to know. The consciousness of a bat is not accessible to humans, but we can assume that bats experience what it is like to be a bat; therefore, we can assume they have a consciousness: "[T]he fact that an organism has conscious experience *at all* means, basically, that there is something that is like to *be* that organism – something it is like *for* the organism" ([5]: 436).

If we follow the research on human consciousness to date, it becomes clear how unclear the answer to the question of its verifiable existence is. A systematic review of theories of consciousness has recently produced a compilation of approximately 30 different theories, some of which are fundamentally contradictory [6]. Furthermore, there has recently been an attempt to find a solution to the problem of consciousness by means of adversarial collaboration. An adversarial collaboration attempts to develop a research design and a subsequent experiment on which researchers with different attitudes have agreed. The experiment should ultimately decide which research group is right. The experiment failed to do so. The authors of the publication on the study concluded: "Most importantly, the debate demonstrated that at this stage, there is more controversy than agreement between the theories, pertaining to the most basic questions of what consciousness is, how to identify conscious states, and what is required from any theory of consciousness" ([7]: 1).

Why is it so difficult to develop a science-based solution to the existence of consciousness? As early as the mid-1990s, the Australian philosopher David Chalmers outlined the question that philosophical and neuroscientific research is still working intensively today, namely, the distinction between the many simple problems and the particularly difficult problem of consciousness research [8]. The particularly "hard" problem, according to Chalmers, is the problem of explaining subjective experience. Put simply, the problem is to understand how the material biological processes of the brain give rise to a feeling or thought that can only be experienced by me. In other words, we cannot explain how my personal experience of a particular colour arises from the synaptic connections of nerve cells during a perceptual process. This is, to use another much-discussed term in philosophy, the *explanatory gap* between matter and the qualities of perceptions that can be experienced only subjectively [9]. These qualities are called, using another philosophical term, *qualia* [10].

What theories have been developed in philosophy and other related scientific disciplines, such as psychology or neuroscience, to solve the "hard problem"? The philosopher Keith Frankish has identified three major theoretical camps, which in turn revolve around the dichotomy of realism and anti-realism [11]. He sees two "realism" camps. First, there are theoretical positions that take the view that there is clearly a human mind but that the explanatory gap or the difficult problem cannot be dealt with scientifically. These include, for example, the philosopher Colin McGinn, who argues that consciousness or the human mind is simply too complicated for us to understand. Consciousness therefore remains a mystery [12]. A second realist position also accepts the explanatory gap but basically assumes that this could be overcome sooner or later on the basis of neuroscience. The core of this position is research into neuronal processes, without which consciousness would not be possible. However, it is currently not possible to explain the transition from biological matter to subjective experience [13].

And then there is a position that at first glance seems quite absurd, but which, from a purely scientific point of view, is—in my opinion—the most convincing theory (for a presentation of this theory that is also accessible to philosophical laypersons, see [14]). This view describes consciousness as an illusion that our brain presents to us [11]. The idea goes back to a proposal by Daniel Dennett, who, in his book *Consciousness Explained* [3] in the early 1990s, called for qualia, i.e. the subjectively perceived properties of perceptions, to be qualified as non-existent. Unlike laypeople in this field, philosophy is not concerned with the question of which approach appears intuitively plausible but which approach is rationally convincing. Illusionism is the approach that is most compatible with a materialistic scientific concept. The "illusion of consciousness" dispenses with the need to explain something that until now has seemed insurmountable as an explanatory gap.

If qualia are regarded as illusions, it is not necessary to explain how they come about. However, it is necessary to explain how the illusion comes about, and this has certainly not yet been fully achieved. One possible explanation is that the illusion of perceiving subjective phenomena has an evolutionary function or at least had one in human history. Daniel Dennett has formulated it as follows: "…consciousness is a user-illusion, a brilliant simplification of the noisy tumult of causation and interaction (at the molecular and cellular levels, for instance) that needs to be prudently and swiftly sampled in order for a brain to do its work of controlling a large complex body through a challenging, changing world" ([15]: 8).

The idea of understanding our psyche or consciousness as an illusion of the brain does not amount to saying that mental illnesses are not real. As the neuroscientist Antonio Damasio recently put it, we cannot simply assume that illusions have no effect [16]. The effect of the illusion of our psyche or consciousness is largely due to cultural influences [17]. In Western culture in particular, we are convinced that we have an individual psyche. This indeed makes us peculiar or odd compared with earlier Western cultures as well as with many non-Western cultures today. The evolutionary biologist Joseph Henrich described this peculiarity with the wonderful acronym WEIRD (*Western, Educated, Industrialised, Rich, Democratic*) [18].

Cultural influences are also used to explain why we are convinced that we have a human psyche, which we experience as essential to who we are as people. In an attempt to unify various theories of consciousness, a team led by neuropsychologist Michael Graziano recently proposed a distinction between information consciousness and mystery consciousness [19]. Information consciousness (*i-consciousness*) is, on one hand, compatible with current neuropsychological theories that explain cognitive processes in particular. Mystery consciousness (*m-consciousness*), on the other hand, goes in the same direction as the theories of illusionism. It refers, for example, to the subjective experience of pain and other qualia phenomena. Although we cannot explain these phenomena scientifically, most cultures and the people associated with them are convinced of the existence of an entity or even an essence that contains such things as psyche, soul or spirit. Such ideas are often described in philosophical research as *folk psychology*, which means something like "everyday psychology". Obviously, we need such attributions in our everyday social lives in order to better understand people and categorise social processes, even if this is not always compatible with science.

I do not expect all readers to follow me and accept the illusionism thesis of consciousness as the best theory in this context. However, it should be clear how much the views on the nature or existence of the psyche, the mind or consciousness differ and where the problems and gaps in explanation lie. From a basic biological perspective—and I can perhaps agree with the sceptics on this—it is therefore completely unclear whether there is a human psyche. The doubts about this are quite pronounced, but we have neither a theoretically sufficient model nor empirical data that could provide more clarity. From my current (!) perspective, our concept of a human psyche can be characterised as a sociocultural attribution of the inner experience of oneself and the behaviour of oneself and others. People in the Global North and West (and many beyond) are convinced of the existence of an individual psyche, and this conviction has probably been brought about more by sociocultural change than by human biology.

However, if this has little or nothing to do with human biology but predominantly with sociocultural developments, then the question naturally arises as to whether coercive measures that are justified by the existence of a disorder of the mind or consciousness could already have problems of argumentation and legitimisation at this abstract level. If we do not know whether people have a biologically based psyche at all, then a central argument in favour of *psychiatric* coercive measures may already fall away here.

5.3   Social Change and Individualisation

Despite the difficulties outlined above in empirically proving or at least defining a human psyche or consciousness, most people in the Global North are convinced of the existence of these phenomena. The following sections have two aims. The first is to reconstruct sociologically and historically why these convictions are so strong that they are not questioned—at least on a broad social level. Second, it is intended to show what exactly is meant by classifying "mental disorders" as sociocultural constructs. The latter argument is intended to contribute to discrediting "mental illness" as a medical basis for legitimising coercive measures in psychiatry.

Social change and the associated attitudes towards oneself and the psyche also remain of central importance for mental illness. Why and for how long have we been convinced that mental illness plays such a major role in our everyday lives and in many other social areas? This major role is all the more astonishing given that psychiatric-epidemiological research almost unanimously assumes that mental disorders or illnesses did not increase in recent decades until the coronavirus pandemic [20–22]. Although there are individual studies that come to different conclusions in certain regions at certain times, systematic reviews and meta-studies show that this is not the case overall.

However, as already indicated, the perception is different. The media, the public and the professional public are largely convinced that mental health problems are increasing in modern society [23]. There are indeed two important indicators that suggest this. First, there has been a significant increase in the use of psychiatric and psychotherapeutic services. An increasing number of people in the Western world and beyond are seeking treatment for mental health problems and are being prescribed appropriate medications such as antidepressants; this is just as much a consensus as the epidemiological facts just mentioned. The second indicator is related to this, namely, that an increasing number of people are taking time off work due to "mental illness". This indicator regularly makes headlines in health insurance reports and gives the impression that there is an increase of "mental illness".

There is no doubt that both phenomena—the non-increase in mental illnesses and the increasing willingness to seek treatment for them—are true. However, how can this be explained? Apparently, mental health problems have been perceived differently in recent decades; they are less taboo and stigmatised. This does not mean that there is no longer any stigma but simply that it is now much less and more differentiated. As recent stigma research has described, certain psychosocial problems, such as depression, are less stigmatised today, whereas others, such as psychoses, are still associated with the desire for distance [24, 25].

Behind this is not only a change in attitudes but also a fundamental social change, which will be briefly outlined below. In the background, we are dealing with a development that sociologists call "functional differentiation" [26]. This, even by historians [27, 28], refers to the fact that modern society is massively influenced by the enforcement of social subsystems such as politics, economics, science, education, law, intimate relationships, etc. These subsystems have been in existence for some time. Although these subsystems had already been established in Western societies since around the eighteenth century, they became widely accepted towards the end of the nineteenth century [29]. This can be seen empirically in the fact that money was only used as a means of payment as part of the economic system in the last village at this time. The same also applies to the state monopoly on the use of force in the political system and the legal system. Prior to this, conflicts had been settled mainly in local milieus.

From a sociological-historical perspective, the subsystems mentioned above have played a key role in the dissolution of traditional social milieus, which we have increasingly experienced since the middle of the twentieth century. Since this time, long-standing working-class and agricultural milieus as well as bourgeois milieus, which had a significant influence on society and the people living in it, have disappeared. Until the 1960s or 1970s, many people still felt that they belonged to these milieus and experienced a corresponding identity. This was evident, for example, in the fact that partners were predominantly chosen from the same milieu and that professional careers were primarily oriented towards those of the parents. In agriculture and mining but also in academically educated milieus, children often followed their parents, particularly with respect to career choices [30].

From today's perspective, the milieus, especially in poorer segments, appear to many observers as positive and community-building. There was certainly some truth in this. However, these milieus were also characterised by poverty, social constriction and control, as well as few opportunities for advancement, exit or development for individuals [31]. In many countries, for example, there was hardly any chance of breaking out of dysfunctional marriages, which particularly affected women. Divorces or abortions were impossible for a long time due to religious and denominational norms, and there were hardly any truly functioning contraceptives.

This all gradually changed from the 1950s and 1960s onwards. Social change was triggered, among other things, by economic development after the Second World War. However, the main driver was the shift from an economic and social structure that was characterised primarily by industry and agriculture to one that was service oriented. Deindustrialisation made itself feel in all Western societies. This was associated with a considerable expansion in education, which allowed for individual advancement and promotion and from which women in particular benefited.

The social structure of Western societies was increasingly characterised by individualisation. It was no longer the social milieus that determined who people married and what profession they took up but rather individual decisions. There were more options available but also many more risks and less standardised lifestyles. With the pressure to make decisions, attention has focused on one's own wishes and sensitivities.

5.4 Individualisation and Psychologisation

In the past, one's own wishes and sensitivities were hardly ever at the centre of decision-making. Decisions were made primarily on the basis of convention, custom, religion and family guidelines. Now, the individual had to see themselves as the centre of action in their own biography, as the sociologist Ulrich Beck aptly formulated in his book *Risk Society* in the 1980s [32]. This required an internal perspective: what do I want to do with my life, how do certain decisions make me feel and how am I doing with my current life? "In the absence of objectifiable criteria of right and wrong, good or evil, the self and its feelings become our only moral guide". This is how Robert N. Bellah and his social science team described the transformation of society and the psyche in the United States at the same time ([33]: 76).

As part of an empirical comparison of the help-seeking behaviour of people in the United States between the 1950s and the 1970s, a research team led by the psychologist Joseph Veroff came to the following conclusion: "It is clear (...) that men and women have become much more psychologically oriented in their thinking about themselves and their lives" ([34]: 38). Empirical indicators of this were the increase in the utilisation of therapeutic services and the decrease in the denial of personal problems.

This development did not please all observers of the time. Philipp Rieff, a conservative American sociologist, was already in the 1970s quick to lament the cultural decline, which, in his view, was associated with the "triumph of the therapeutic". According to his analysis, with the establishment of the market and democracy, religious authorities and customs lost their cultural character. "The religious man was born to be saved; psychological man was born to be pleased" ([35]: 19). Rieff saw a certain necessity in the transition from religion to therapy, as human existence in modern society did not produce inner peace with itself, as was the case—according to his conviction—with religiously characterised culture. Rieff was not alone in this criticism, and it did not only come from the conservative side. In the 1970s, sociologist Christopher Lasch, for example, lamented a "culture of narcissism" that was associated with excessive individualism and an accompanying "popularisation of psychiatric modes of thought" ([36]: 25).

This complex of changing cultural practices, such as the increasing use of psychotherapy and changing ways of thinking, is currently described in sociology with the term psychologisation [37]. However, the effects of psychologisation go far beyond these aspects. Psychological semantics can be found in almost every sector of society today. The entire field of education is based on psychological thinking, and the legal system examines many questions from a psychological perspective (e.g. when determining culpability); in the media, you cannot avoid relevant articles or advice programmes and our everyday working life (e.g. when recruiting employees through assessment centres), or our everyday relationships are hardly imaginable without psychological references ("What are you feeling about that?").

5.5 Interaction of Sensitivities and Diagnostic Classifications

Overall, it should be noted that psychological sensitivities are receiving much more attention today than they did in previous generations. This fact is undisputed. The increased attention given to mental health and the utilisation of therapeutic services has consequences that must be assessed ambivalently. On the one hand, it is certainly positive that the stigma of mental illness and psychiatric or psychotherapeutic measures has decreased considerably in recent decades. Today, it is no longer shameful to admit to being treated for depression or an anxiety disorder—it is a different story with psychoses or addiction disorders. On the other hand, however, increased awareness of one's own psyche contributes to a feeling of emotional vulnerability [38]. We experience our everyday lives to a large extent from the perspective of psychological or emotional stress.

As we increasingly seek medical or therapeutic help for mental health problems, we are also more frequently confronted with corresponding diagnoses. Diagnostic classification systems such as the DSM or the ICD, whose weaknesses will be discussed later, play a central role in the provision of help, be it medication or psychotherapy. No health insurance will pay without a diagnosis. Our problems are therefore not only psychologised but also medicalised; i.e. private or social problems are transformed and reinterpreted as medical issues [39]. This mechanism can be used to illustrate the phenomenon of reification, which is known from philosophy and will be explained in more detail later. The diagnostic classifications provide professionals and laypersons with their precise criteria for individual disorders. These criteria are classified as "true", and all those involved, as well as the media and other subsystems of society, such as education or the legal system, adopt the characteristics of their programmes or their decisions. The more often this

5.5 Interaction of Sensitivities and Diagnostic Classifications

mechanism is repeated, the more convinced professionals, sufferers and the general public are of the existence of the disorders. There is no pharmaceutical industry conspiracy behind medicalisation, even if the pharmaceutical industry contributes in some detail. It is the repeated communication and application of certain criteria that unfolds its effect and creates its own "reality" of mental disorders.

This medicalisation plays a significant role in how we experience and define our mental states. An increasing number of areas of everyday life are being medicalised and, in the psychiatric field, are being psychologised. A few years ago, social scientists Allan Horwitz and Jerome Wakefield focused on how previously non-medicalised issues such as grief reactions were labelled depression during changes to classification systems. The book was aptly titled *The Loss of Sadness* [40]. A few years later, this development prompted the main author of the DSM-IV, Allen Frances, to write a critical book about the entire development of the classifications, which was also aptly titled *Saving Normal* [41].

Our everyday problems are therefore defined to a significant extent by psychologisation and medicalisation, which changes the way we experience them. In the Western world, we hardly notice this anymore, as we have presumably become accustomed to these processes and medicalisation does have positive aspects. Just think of the decriminalisation of drug use. However, medicalisation and psychologisation are also being exported to many non-Western regions, with the diagnostic and statistical manual (DSM) and the international classification of diseases (ICD) becoming quasi-standards for diagnosis. Interestingly, this changes the perception of problems. One particular aspect of this is "hyperintrospection", i.e. the massively increased focus on one's own well-being. This form of psychologisation is not only found in the Global North but also in many regions of the Global South ([42]: 254).

It may seem that our experience of problems is shaped exclusively by medicalisation, psychologisation and classification systems. However, this is not the case. There is also another direction, namely, that social movements influence diagnostic systems. Two prominent examples in recent decades were the removal of the diagnosis "homosexuality" from the DSM, which was still officially categorised as a mental disorder until 1980, and the inclusion of 'post-traumatic stress disorder' (PTSD) in the DSM following massive pressure from US Vietnam War veterans. The latter initiative had not only therapeutic motivation but also a clear political background. It "...was driven by the idea that an immoral war had done serious psychological damage to its participants" ([43]: 93). The topic of psychotrauma received a great deal of attention through its inclusion in the DSM from 1980 onwards and would certainly not be recognised and considered to the same extent today if this had not happened. Research on PTSD began only in the 1980s and 1990s.

This should clarify what interactions exist between the mental state of the population and the classification systems. Classification systems define the details of psychological sensitivities, and these sensitivities have an effect on classification systems in certain variations. The Canadian philosopher and historian of science, Ian Hacking, characterised this as a "looping effect". "People classified in a certain way tend to conform or to grow into the ways they are described; but they also evolve in their own ways, so that the classifications and descriptions have to be constantly revised" ([44]: 21). That is, classifications and sensitivities are in a constant state of flux of mutual influence and change. Hacking came across this fact when he tried to explain why certain "mental illnesses", such as hysteria, fugue or multiple personality disorder, were very prevalent at certain times and then disappeared almost completely. The "illnesses" came and disappeared not only from the medical-therapeutic perspective but also in the real lives of the patients.

From a sociological perspective, "mental illnesses" are therefore the result of a combination of social change, changes in attitudes in the population and medical classifications. These phenomena are demonstrably subject to considerable sociocultural influences. Even the inclusion or exclusion of diagnoses in classification systems—as seen in the context of PTSD and homosexuality—was not a purely medical decision.

5.6 Mentally "Ill" or "Not Ill": Historical Developments Between Eugenics and Psychiatry

Since our ideas about the human psyche have been shaped by cultural factors, the same applies to our prevailing beliefs about what constitutes a mental illness. But what does this look like from a medical or psychological perspective? To explore this question, I leave sociology behind. I turn to aspects that every person working in psychiatry and probably many people affected by psychiatric care will have asked themselves. The key question is as follows: How can we distinguish what we call "mental illness" from non-illness? In the relevant research literature, this is described with the term *boundary problem* or *demarcation problem* [45, 46]. Related to this are further problems, such as the following: What criteria do we use to define the boundary between sick and healthy?

These questions have preoccupied psychiatric and psychological research since its beginnings. What is normal, and what is not in connection with human characteristics? Terms such as "abnormal" are still used today in connection with psychological characteristics. The term "abnormal" emerged in the mid-nineteenth century and has persisted to the present day, although "hereditary abnormality" was the central focus of eugenics during National Socialism, which led first to sterilisation and then to the murder of hundreds of thousands of people with intellectual and psychosocial problems. The "hereditary abnormalities" included "schizophrenia", "manic-depressive psychosis", "severe psychopathy", "hysteria", "homosexuality", "drug addiction" and "alcoholism" [47]. The *Journal of Abnormal Psychology* changed its name to *Journal of Psychopathology and Clinical Science* as late as 2022. Textbooks with corresponding titles are also still available today [48].

In my opinion, the inglorious contributions of early statistics and early psychology to eugenics, which are associated with the names Francis Galton (normal distribution), Karl Pearson (correlation coefficient) or Ronald A. Fisher (maximum likelihood estimation method) [49], are among the facts of scientific history that are not sufficiently known. The concepts and methods mentioned in the brackets are still part of the basics of statistics today and are taught at every university. Interestingly, the concept of the "normal" was first developed through statistics, and it was only in the course of the twentieth century that it became popularised to the extent that it became part of everyday language. The "normal distribution" was, as the relevant historical research has worked out, the decisive development for the idea that the average must also be healthy [50]. The idea of the "normal" and the "abnormal" is just as characterised by sociocultural developments as the idea of "mental disorder". This applies not only to psychology or psychiatry but also to almost all fields of medicine and topics such as sexual orientation.

In recent psychiatric history, however, this has fundamentally changed, and many clinicians are still convinced that "mental disorders" are clearly definable disease entities that are abnormal conditions. These beliefs date back to the 1970s, when considerable efforts were made, particularly in US psychiatry, to turn psychiatry into a medical field that was essentially no different from other fields. First, this was a reaction to the anti-psychiatric movement, which included the psychiatrist Thomas Szasz, the philosopher Michel Foucault and the sociologists Erving Goffman and Thomas Scheff, among others. What these authors have in common is the conviction that social and cultural factors are formative, if not decisive, for the perception of "mental illness".

Second, the "scientific nature" of psychiatry was heavily criticised, especially after the so-called Rosenhan experiment, in which feigned psychiatric symptoms led to admissions to US hospitals. This experiment, the publication of which even made it into an academic publication flagship *Science* [51], was widely regarded as proof of the unscientific approach of psychiatry. We now know that David Rosenhan himself used highly questionable procedures in his experiments that call his academic integrity into question [52]. Interestingly, the reactions of the academic psychiatry community in the United States have gone in two directions. On the one hand, the fundamental criticism of Rosenhan and his scientific methodology was rejected. On the other hand, this criticism was taken as evidence that scientific procedures should now be introduced to improve the reliability of diagnoses [53], i.e. to ensure that symptoms from different practitioners are reliably assigned to the same diagnoses.

The intention to make psychiatry a medical speciality like all others culminated in a publication by Gerald Klerman [54], then President of the National Alcohol and Drug Abuse and Mental Health Authority (ADAMHA). In a kind of manifesto, the following theses, among others, were proposed:

> (1) Psychiatry is a branch of medicine. (2) Psychiatry should utilize modern scientific methodologies and base its practice on scientific knowledge. (3) Psychiatry treats people who are ill and need treatment for mental illness. (4) There is a boundary between the normal and the sick. (5) There are discrete mental illnesses. Mental illnesses are not myths. There is not one but many mental illnesses. (...) (6) The focus of the psychiatric physician should be particularly on the biological aspects of mental illness. (...) ([54]: 104)

Klerman used the example of schizophrenia to illustrate the concept of illness later in the publication. In his view, certain experiences and behaviours are classified as abnormal. Although there is a certain correspondence with the emotional life of 'normal people', the intensity, duration and extent of the disorder suggest that all of this should be categorised as an illness.

5.7 The Problem of Demarcation

An important example from the 1970s also shows how difficult the solutions are and how (it must be said at the end) arbitrary the definition of boundaries is. The so-called Feighner criteria were an instrument in the development of modern classification systems at this time. As with later versions of the US diagnostic manual DSM, the boundary between the diagnosis and non-diagnosis of a particular disorder was drawn on the basis of the number of symptoms. This approach went back to studies in the 1950s, where it was determined, for example, that six out of ten symptoms had to be present for a diagnosis of depression. Decades later, when one of the authors was asked why six out of ten, he replied: "It sounded about right" ([55]: 136). This rather arbitrary practice was retained in later versions of the Feighner criteria. Central criteria continue to be set according to clinical judgement and not on the basis of empirical studies.

The current definition of mental disorders in the ICD-11 version of the WHO disease classification, which came into force at the beginning of 2022, is as follows: "Mental, behavioural and neurodevelopmental disorders are syndromes characterised by clinically significant disturbance in an individual's cognition, emotional regulation, or behaviour that reflects a dysfunction in the psychological, biological, or developmental processes that underlie mental and behavioural functioning. These disturbances are usually associated with distress or impairment in personal, family, social, educational, occupational, or other important areas of functioning" [56].

This rather complex and not readily understandable definition is a good illustration of where the problems lie with drawing boundaries and the associated criteria. First, clinical significance is emphasised, i.e. the assessment of professionals regarding the extent of a phenomenon. Second, dysfunction in psychological or biological processes is postulated. Ideally, this involves objectifiable dysfunctions in the brain or in mental processes that must be related to the clinical assessment. Third, it is about the experience of stress and impairments that should be noticeable in the everyday life of the person affected.

Clinical significance describes obvious disease characteristics that, for specialists, represent a clear deviation from healthy conditions. These signs are usually defined using classification systems such as the ICD. A severe depressive episode is indicated, for example, by a significantly lowered mood, reduced interest in everyday activities, concentration problems or feelings of worthlessness. Boundary-drawing problems are recognisable in regard to describing the level at which one can speak of a lowered mood, when an interest in everyday activities should be considered reduced or how pronounced feelings of worthlessness should be to assign them clinical significance. It is to be expected that clinical significance will be determined by comparison with "normal" or "healthy" reference classes.

5.7 The Problem of Demarcation

However, the validity and reliability of these findings are not particularly strong because we do not know what "normal" and "healthy" actually mean.

Even more problematic, however, is the reference to mental or biological processes that are supposed to be dysfunctional. As there are no valid biomarkers for corresponding dysfunctions, the clinician is again reliant on observations and interview results that are hypothetically supposed to establish links to mental processes. Even if such markers are to exist at some point, which is not particularly likely, the issue of demarcation will arise with regard to what corresponds to the norm and what does not. In addition, no less problematic in terms of drawing boundaries is the reference to stresses or impairments in social relationships or other areas of everyday life. Where for example, should the line be drawn in terms of the number or intensity of social contacts? In the area of work or education, a significant number of days off work can lead to difficulties. However, where is the line drawn between acceptable and unacceptable numbers?

Interestingly, the ICD-11 describes conditions for the diagnoses that are labelled as "limits to normality (threshold)". For the diagnosis of schizophrenia (code 6A20), for example, psychotic experiences or symptoms may occur in the general population but are "... usually transient in nature and not accompanied by other symptoms of schizophrenia or deterioration in psychosocial functioning" (http://id.who.int/icd/entity/1683919430; 10.12.2022). In the case of affective disorders, depression is described as a normal reaction to certain negative life events but differs from these in terms of "severity, extent and duration" (http://id.who.int/icd/entity/76398729; 10.12.2022). On the one hand, these attempts at differentiation are certainly important and commendable, but on the other hand, the arbitrariness and individual assessment of professionals become clear, which affects not only validity but also reliability.

How does psychiatric research address this problem? Generally, there are two different camps. On the one hand, there is the biological or naturalistic camp. In this camp, physical indicators are sought that should at least help to distinguish more clearly between sick and healthy individuals. On the other hand, there is the values camp. This is not primarily concerned with which criteria we can use to determine what is ill and what is not ill. This camp tends to focus on analysing how social values or constructs shape the views that make people appear mentally ill.

Within the biological camp, there are three major approaches. The "classic" approach is the biostatistical theory of Christopher Boorse [57]. Here, health and disease are related to a comparable group of organisms or people. Health refers to the typical characteristics of this group that it needs for its members to survive and reproduce. The theory itself requires that no social values be involved. However, this cannot be upheld, as the relevant research literature has established [45]. The fact that these characteristics can also be influenced by social values becomes clear with respect to sexual orientation. Homosexual orientations, for example, are, in many cases, contrary to human reproduction and can be classified as a disorder in this theory.

The second approach is the *harmful dysfunction* concept by social scientist Jerome Wakefield [58]. Here, on the one hand, an even stronger reference to evolutionary theory is postulated, and on the other hand, the surrounding culture of the person affected is emphasised. A mental disorder is therefore based on functions selected during human development, which manifest themselves as dysfunction in everyday life. It therefore requires a biological basis that has a detrimental effect on a person's social functioning. Wakefield's approach is now considered the quasi-standard in the clinical definition of mental disorders, as we find them in the DSM and ICD classifications [59]. However, this approach was criticised early on [60] and is still controversial today [61]. Central points of discussion are the postulate that biopsychological dysfunctions have been evolutionarily selected, the problem of functionality and dysfunctionality (which I will discuss in general below), and finally, the difficulty of drawing a clear boundary, which Wakefield also acknowledges. In his view, however, the latter is not a fundamental problem, as the particularly striking outlier value would be considered an indicator of a disorder [62].

Third, the aforementioned biomarkers as characteristics have been used as a basis for the biological camp in recent years. The idea behind biomarkers is to postulate laboratory- or imaging-based findings as clear evidence of disease. A biomarker is a "...characteristic that is objectively measured and evaluated as an indicator of normal biological processes, pathogenic processes or pharmacological responses to a therapeutic intervention" ([63]: 91). This approach is used to model Alzheimer's dementia, where certain indicators can be detected in the cerebrospinal fluid. However, it has not yet been possible to find such clear biomarkers for mental disorders, which are very complex in their development. One of the fundamental problems is the still necessary reference to nonbiological symptoms to determine disease relevance [64], as standard findings for mental disorders do not exist biologically and probably never will.

The biomarker problem is also one of the reasons why the current classification systems in psychiatry, such as the DSM or the ICD, are being called into question by biological research in psychiatry. In biological research, the criteria for "illness" formulated in classification systems are not particularly helpful. There are hardly any connections, let alone causal connections, between biological characteristics and the criteria formulated in the classifications. Instead of these, usually artificially drawn demarcations, biological research favours a dimensional concept in which the characteristics are continuously distributed [65].

However, there is a great deal of doubt as to whether this approach provides a better solution to the fundamental problem of drawing boundaries. Robert Plomin, one of the best-known and most important behavioural genetics researchers, recently presented an analysis of this issue from a genetic perspective. According to this analysis, the characteristics that are used for mental disorders do not differ qualitatively but rather differ purely quantitatively from non-diseased conditions. "Genetic research shows that the medical model is all wrong when it comes to psychological problems. What we call disorders are merely the extremes of the same genes work throughout the normal distribution" ([66]: 58). His conclusion: "Abnormal is normal". In other words, from a basic biological perspective, it is not possible to make a meaningful distinction between ill and well.

5.8 The Problem of Psychological Dysfunction

Now, for the values camp [67, 68]. Here, the problem of drawing boundaries is usually seen as an attempt to classify normative characteristics in terms of social deviation or deviance as "sick" and to ensure that people labelled in this way receive psychiatric treatment—possibly even against their will. The history of psychiatry is full of examples that cannot be dismissed. These range from the supposedly pathological urge of slaves in the United States to flee their situation ("drapetomania") to the aforementioned treatment of same-sex relationships, which appeared as a diagnosis in the DSM-III diagnostic manual until 1980. In addition, it has not disappeared even today, for example, in the ICD-11. Although exclusively moral judgements are not considered sufficient for a psychiatric diagnosis, they still play a central role, as the following description of "disorder with compulsive sexual behaviour (code 6C72)" shows: "Symptoms may include repetitive sexual activities becoming a central focus of the person's life to the point of neglecting health and personal care or other interests, activities and responsibilities; numerous unsuccessful efforts to significantly reduce repetitive sexual behavior; and continued repetitive sexual behavior despite adverse consequences or deriving little or no satisfaction from it."

In the official classifications of the ICD and DSM, deviation or deviance is naturally excluded. For formal reasons alone, social judgements do not belong to a disease concept. The substitute term is again dysfunction. Dysfunction has already been mentioned above in connection with Wakefield's model of harm-related dysfunction, which is based on evolutionary theory. However, current classifications do not go that far but define dysfunction in connection with the experience of stress and disability [69]. The idea behind this is, for example, that too much alcohol consumption has a dysfunctional effect on health and that a depressive mood has a negative impact not only on physical health but also on social relationships or that, as cited in the example above, "compulsive sexual behaviour" can lead to neglect of personal hygiene.

In this way, social and normative judgements are introduced into the dysfunction through the back door. What stresses a person and what makes them feel disabled is not solely dependent on psychological phenomena but also on how the social environment sees and reacts to them. Why should a young man not be allowed to neglect personal hygiene in favour of, for example, permanent porn consumption and masturbation? Even if this should not be tolerated by his environment and he neglects responsibilities by not going to school or not working, what makes this behavioural complex a pathological behaviour as long as he himself does not suffer from it? Is it not rather the case that "That's not the way it should be…" that plays a central role here?

Incidentally, the relevance of evaluations from the social environment does not apply only to psychological phenomena. To stay in the field of sexuality, so-called erectile dysfunction is a fairly widespread phenomenon that does not occur only with increasing age. From a purely biological point of view, dysfunction can be defined as a lack of or insufficient erection under sexual stimulation. In a sexual relationship, however, the lack of an erection only becomes dysfunctional when it has a negative effect on the relationship and possibly causes distress. However, if satisfactory erotic behaviour is developed for all parties involved or if certain forms of sexuality are completely avoided with the consent of all parties involved, then it is no longer a dysfunction.

This is the same with respect to psychological phenomena. Even from a neuroscientific perspective, it is now recognised that psychological problems arise from the combination of the dimensional characteristics of a certain trait and the respective environment: "Sometimes we might have extreme values in one dimension, but the extent to which that value is *problematic* depends a lot of other factors, including our environments" ([70]: 15). According to this perspective, "normality" is a mixture of typical and functional characteristics. Both the typical and the functional are interspersed with normative social judgements.

In a social environment that reacts much more tolerantly to drug use, hallucinations or mood swings, people with these phenomena feel less burdened or even handicapped. Social normative judgements cannot be avoided in this context [71]: Why should not I drink more than my environment allows me to drink? Why should not I be allowed to be in a bad mood? Why should not I have more sex or less sex than is generally considered normal? Dysfunctions or deficits are, as was recently established in a corresponding analysis from the autism field, "neurocognitive differences in neurotypical environments" [72]. It is the "typical" social environment that determines what constitutes a deficit or dysfunction. The concept of neurodiversity will be presented in more detail in the following chapter.

The concept of disability in particular has recently been defined primarily in social terms. The United Nations Convention on the Rights of Persons with Disabilities, which has already been mentioned several times, is explicitly based—as described in Chap. 2—on a social model that no longer sees the reason for disability in the person but rather on the environment that hinders the exercise of participation by the person [73]. In connection with physical disabilities, the environment is already being designed in many places so that people with wheelchairs can make better use of public transport, for example, by installing lifts at railway stations or making buses easier to access. This is not readily apparent in the case of psychosocial problems. This would mean designing social environments in such a way that the people affected are better included. Rehabilitation programmes such as Supported Employment or Supported Housing provide for precisely this purpose [74]. But then of course the question arises: if the environment is optimised, is the affected person still disabled in terms of their ability to function? And what does this mean for the diagnosis of a mental disorder?

What does all this mean for the question of whether we can make a clear distinction between "mentally healthy" and "mentally ill"? On the basis of the state of research reported here, it should have become clear that this is hardly possible. In this respect, it is not surprising that recent publications on this topic use terms such as "vague" or "fuzzy" to characterise the problem of drawing boundaries between sick and healthy individuals in psychiatry [75]. The former president of the largest US research institute in psychiatry, Steve Hyman, summarised the consequences as follows: "The boundaries between ill and well require policy decisions with respect to setting thresholds, as is the case in all of medicine, for disorders that represent quantitative deviations from health" ([76]: 23). In pointing out the fundamental problem in medicine, Hyman is indeed right. This problem does not affect psychiatry alone but can be found in many medical specialties [77]. What is special about psychiatry, however, is that the people affected may be given a diagnosis against their will, placed in an institution against their will and often treated involuntarily. This makes this topic a particular professional and ethical challenge, which is not the same as the question of where to draw the line on hypertension or diabetes mellitus. A risk to one's own health in the context of diabetes, which is known to be not uncommon, does not result in coercive measures, whereas a risk to one's own health in the context of a diagnosed depressive disorder does.

5.9 Can a Distinction Be Made Between Different Mental Disorders?

Psychiatric classification systems and the diagnoses they describe have various purposes. In practical terms, they are intended to provide clinical professionals and service users with clarity about various clinical pictures, to facilitate communication between professionals and users and, last but not least, to enable billing with cost bearers. From a scientific point of view, they should provide clear definitions and criteria that allow research to be conducted into causes or treatment options. The core of classification systems lies in the description of the numerous different clinical pictures, for example, the establishment of criteria for characterising a depressive disorder as distinct from an anxiety disorder.

In medicine in general, and therefore also in psychiatry, such classification systems are regularly revised to fulfil the requirement that new scientific findings are reflected in a differentiated way in the descriptions of mental disorders. This naturally also applies to the DSM and the ICD, which are regularly revised. The revision of the DSM-IV classification to the DSM-5, which was introduced in 2013, was associated with many hopes on the part of both clinical and research professionals to address the numerous weaknesses. One of the weaknesses was the difficulty in distinguishing between ill and non-ill, as mentioned in the previous section. It was generally agreed that a categorical system was of little use in doing justice given the complexity of mental health problems. Instead, a continuous and dimensional system should be developed [78]. In the end, however, a categorical system was established again, which is better suited for legal and reimbursement purposes than dimensionality.

In addition to categorisation, the validity of the clinical pictures and their criteria was a major topic of discussion. In this context, validity refers to the question of whether the descriptive features actually reflect an underlying clinical picture. Modern psychiatric classification systems are structured a-theoretically, i.e. they do not—formally speaking—reflect a specific model of mental disorders but describe particular characteristics and behaviours. This was a reaction to the early systems, which were primarily psychodynamic in nature. Since the introduction of the DSM-III in 1980, however, the classifications have aimed to improve agreement between professionals regarding individual disorders. Validity was neglected in favour of so-called interrater reliability. Interrater reliability is a measure of the agreement between different professionals who, for example, examine and interview a patient and then come to an assessment of the diagnosis. In the early classification systems, agreement was relatively low, which made the psychiatric systems appear dubious and unscientific.

It is therefore hardly surprising that biological research, of all things, has little favour for the DSM/ICD system. As already mentioned, there are few associations between biological factors and markers and the characteristics described in the classification systems. From a biological point of view, the diagnoses are not very valid, i.e. the schizophrenia characteristics only reflect the biological findings to a limited extent. Not least for this reason, an initiative was founded a few years ago to generate new research criteria for psychopathology. Funded by the US National Institute of Mental Health (NIMH), the *Research Domain Criteria* (RDoC) project aims at nothing less than a new basis for psychopathology [79]. Instead of the usual behavioural patterns and observations, so-called endophenotypes are now to be researched, i.e. primarily markers that should ideally represent biological or neuropsychological dysfunctions.

In contrast to the categorical diagnoses, RDoC describes six domains that are intended to redefine psychopathology as a whole: negative valence, positive valence, cognitive systems, systems for social processes, systems of arousal and regulation and sensorimotor systems [80]. Across various biological and psychological areas, the aim is to describe new relationships and thus create impulses for the—primarily biological—causal research of mental illnesses. Conventional diagnostic categorisations are declared obsolete, as RDoC believes that they both artificially separate similarities between differently viewed disorders and make differences in standardised diagnostic groups invisible. In other words, RDoC abolishes the diagnoses that have been established for many decades, at least from a research perspective.

Another initiative with similar aims is the HiTOP system. HiTOP stands for "Hierarchical Taxonomy of Psychopathology" [81]. On the basis of statistical analyses of symptoms and syndromes, six spectra have been defined that are to be considered dimensionally. Specifically, according to the latest version of the taxonomy, these are the following spectra: Somatoform, Internalisation, Thought Disorder, Detachment, Disinhibited Externalisation, and Antagonistic Externalisation [82]. The authors of the HiTOP approach hope that this comparatively very reduced framework will provide both clearer causal relationships and better clinical benefits.

The "p-factor" approach is even more reduced. Analogous to the g-factor of general intelligence, this approach assumes only one factor, namely, general psychopathology. Empirically, the P-factor is based on the "Dunedin study", which is particularly well-known in developmental psychology. This is a longitudinal cohort study from New Zealand in which a birth cohort was followed over several decades and repeatedly re-examined [83]. The researchers have reported a high degree of comorbidity of various disorders in the life course of people affected by mental health problems, which has raised considerable doubts about the diversity of the problem situations. They suspect a general susceptibility ("liability"), which is ultimately unspecific but can trigger cognitive difficulties in particular [84].

In summary, it is clear that, from the point of view of basic research, there are considerable doubts about the clinical pictures that we have thought we have known for a long time and that many specialists and many people in the population are convinced that they exist. The concept of mental illness has a triple problem of demarcation. First, it is not possible to distinguish between different types of disorders clearly. Second, it is not possible to make a clear distinction between symptoms and non-symptomatic characteristics. Finally, and most importantly, it is not possible to make a clear distinction between dysfunction and function, i.e. between ill and well.

From a research perspective, the fact that we have relied on interrater reliability and lost sight of validity and possible causes is obviously now taking its toll. To a certain extent, the diagnoses of the DSM and ICD classification systems have taken on a life of their own, a circumstance known in the philosophy of science as "reification" [85]. This means that the concept of a certain issue becomes so powerful that it reifies itself. Professionals and many users have assigned symptoms to diagnoses for decades and are ultimately convinced that depression is seen as being just as present as a cancer-causing tumour. From a research perspective, however, it is clear that mental disorders are not like tumours; rather, they are not natural disease entities. It is relatively certain that mental disorders or illnesses are not *natural kinds*, which exist independently of our conceptual constructs, but rather *practical kinds*, i.e. pragmatically selected entities that appear useful from a clinical perspective [86].

In view of this situation, it must be stated that we are not much further than "I know it when I see it..." with regard to a valid definition and differentiation of individual mental illnesses from other illnesses and non-ill conditions. This famous sentence by a judge of the United States Supreme Court made legal history when it came to defining pornography in 1964. In his opinion on the question of whether a Louis Malle film, now classified as a classic, should not be shown in cinemas, he remarked that he would not even attempt to draw up a definition in view of the problems. However, he knew what pornography was when he saw it, and the film did not fall under the pornography criteria [87]. This was just as pragmatic a description as usual for mental disorders in everyday clinical practice. And just like "mental disorders", the definition of pornography is still ambiguous and controversial [88].

5.10 Conclusion: Human Rights and the Real Construct of Mental Disorder

As already described at the beginning, Thomas Szasz became known in the early 1960s with the thesis that mental illness was a myth [89]. Szasz primarily saw the reason for this in the fact that mental illnesses could not be proven to be biological defects. From today's perspective, it must be stated that biology has been able to clarify much that is relevant to the pathology of the psyche—if we know exactly what the pathology of the psyche means. Today, we know much more about the causes that lead to different experiences and behaviours in people. However, we cannot say exactly what "psyche" means, and we also cannot say exactly what "pathological" means.

Does this mean that mental illness is a myth in the sense of Thomas Szasz? In my view, that is not correct. It is not a myth, i.e. something that does not exist. In philosophy, there are two major camps with regard to these topics: realism and that of anti-realism [1]. Realist positions assume the existence of mental illness; anti-realist positions deny this.

I am a realist; I am convinced that mental illnesses exist but probably not in the sense in which they are usually thought of. Most of what we associate with mental phenomena are sociocultural constructs. This starts with the construct of emotion. For a long time, people were convinced that there were universal biological emotions such as fear or anger, which are expressed similarly to reactions in every culture. Today, however, current neuroscientific research sees emotion as a culturally dependent construct that is not a reaction but rather a kind of prediction and expectation function of the brain. However, according to emotion researcher Lisa Feldman Barrett in her fundamental work on the subject, this does not mean that these emotions are not "real": "The distinction between 'real in nature' versus 'illusory' is a false dichotomy. Fear and anger are real to a group of people who *agree* that certain changes in the body on the face are meaningful as emotions. In other words, emotion concepts have a *social reality*" ([90]: 133).

I see the significance of "mental illness" in a very similar way. On the biological level, we find no hard evidence for mental illness in the sense of valid definitions of "psyche" and "illness" but rather considerable ambiguities (consciousness, etc.) and dimensional manifestations of biological characteristics. However, most people are convinced of the existence of mental illness, which suggests that the concept should be seen as a social construct. To take up Lisa Feldman Barrett's argument, social constructs are absolutely real and have very real consequences.

Many readers may not even realise how much social constructs dominate our society. However, this can be illustrated quite simply via the example of money. Cash, fiat money or, more recently to a certain extent, cryptocurrencies function on the basis of social trust that an equivalent value is associated with them. Since money is no longer tied to gold, however, countervalue has become a purely social construct that works perfectly well. However, people can also decide to do without money as a medium of exchange. This makes life much more arduous, but it is conceivable to manage on a self-sufficient farm without money. It is the same as the social construct of mental illness. It is a widely recognised social construct but one that depends on the agreement of the people involved, as noted above. That said, I as a person can choose not to, and there is no valid argument to necessarily convince me of the existence of mental disorders or illness.

And it is these uncertainties that, in my view, do not justify psychiatrically treating people against their will. In both acute psychiatry and forensic psychiatry, the identification of a mental disorder is a necessary prerequisite for forcibly hospitalising people and, under certain circumstances, treating them. However, if we do not know exactly what a mental disorder is, if it can be assumed that sociocultural aspects are more important than medical criteria and if we do not even truly know about the existence of the human psyche, then I am convinced that an essential argument for justifying the use of coercion, i.e. the medically legitimised violation of human rights, no longer applies.

References

1. Graham G. The disordered mind: an introduction to philosophy of mind and mental illness. 2nd ed. Londen/New York: Routledge; 2013.
2. Richter D. Psychisches System und soziale Umwelt: Soziologie psychischer Störungen in der Ära der Biowissenschaften. Bonn: Psychiatrie-Verlag; 2003.
3. Dennett D. Consciousness explained. Boston: Little, Brown and Co.; 1991.
4. Koch C. The quest for consciousness: a neurobiological approach. Englewood: Roberts and Company; 2004.
5. Nagel T. What is it like to be a bat? Philos Rev. 1974;83(4):435–50.
6. Seth AK, Bayne T. Theories of consciousness. Nat Rev Neurosci. 2022;23(7):439–52.
7. Mudrik L, Boly M, Dehaene S, Fleming SM, Lamme V, Seth A, et al. Unpacking the complexities of consciousness: theories and reflections. Neurosci Biobehav Rev. 2025;170:106053.
8. Chalmers DJ. Facing up to the problem of consciousness. J Conscious Stud. 1995;2(3):200–19.
9. Levine J. Materialism and qualia: the explanatory gap. Pac Philos Q. 1983;64(4):354–61.
10. Block N. Qualia. In: Guttenplan S, editor. A companion to the philosophy of mind. Oxford: Blackwell; 1994. p. 514–20.
11. Frankish K. Illusionism as a theory of consciousness. J Conscious Stud. 2016;23(11–12):11–39.
12. McGinn C. The mysterious flame: conscious minds in a material world. New York: Basic Books; 1999.
13. Frith CD. The neural basis of consciousness. Psychol Med. 2021;51(4):550–62.
14. Frankish K. The consciousness illusion; 2019. Available from: https://aeon.co/essays/what-if-your-consciousness-is-an-illusion-created-by-your-brain
15. Dennett DC. A history of qualia. Topoi. 2020;39(1):5–12.
16. Damasio A. The strange order of things: life, feeling, and the making of cultures. New York: Pantheon; 2019.
17. Humphrey N. Soul dust: the magic of consciousness. Princeton: Princeton University Press; 2011.
18. Henrich J. The WEIRDest people in the world: how the west became psychologically peculiar and particularly prosperous. London: Penguin; 2020.
19. Graziano MSA, Guterstam A, Bio BJ, Wilterson AI. Toward a standard model of consciousness: reconciling the attention schema, global workspace, higher-order thought, and illusionist theories. Cogn Neuropsychol. 2020;37(3–4):155–72.
20. GBD Disease Injury IP. Global, regional, and national incidence, prevalence, and years lived with disability for 354 diseases and injuries for 195 countries and territories, 1990-2017: a systematic analysis for the global burden of disease study 2017. Lancet. 2018;392(10159):1789–858.
21. Baxter AJ, Scott KM, Ferrari AJ, Norman RE, Vos T, Whiteford HA. Challenging the myth of an "epidemic" of common mental disorders: trends in the global prevalence of anxiety and depression between 1990 and 2010. Depress Anxiety. 2014;31(6):506–16.
22. Richter D, Wall A, Bruen A, Whittington R. Is the global prevalence rate of adult mental illness increasing? Systematic review and meta-analysis. Acta Psychiatr Scand. 2019;140(5):393–407.
23. Richter D. Die vermeintliche Zunahme psychischer Erkrankungen – Gesellschaftlicher Wandel und psychische Gesundheit. Psychiatr Prax. 2020;47(7):349–51.
24. Pescosolido BA, Halpern-Manners A, Luo L, Perry B. Trends in public stigma of mental illness in the US, 1996-2018. JAMA Netw Open. 2021;4(12):e2140202.

25. Schomerus G, Schindler S, Sander C, Baumann E, Angermeyer MC. Changes in mental illness stigma over 30 years – improvement, persistence, or deterioration? Eur Psychiatry. 2022;65(1):e78.
26. Luhmann N. Die Gesellschaft der Gesellschaft. Frankfurt/M: Suhrkamp; 1997.
27. Rödder A. 21.0 – Eine kurze Geschichte der Gegenwart. München: Beck; 2015.
28. Ziemann B. Gesellschaft ohne Zentrum: Deutschland in der differenzierten Moderne. Ditzingen: Reclam; 2024.
29. Richter D. Nation als form. Wiesbaden: Westdeutscher Verlag; 1996.
30. Raphael L. Jenseits von Kohle und Stahl: Eine Gesellschaftsgeschichte Westeuropas nach dem Boom. Frankfurt/M: Suhrkamp; 2019.
31. Lawrence J. Me Me Me? The search for community in post-war England. Oxford: Oxford University Press; 2019.
32. Beck U. Risikogesellschaft: Auf dem Weg in eine andere Moderne. Frankfurt M: Suhrkamp Verlag; 1986.
33. Bellah RN, Madsen R, Sullivan WM, Swidler A, Tipton SM. Habits of the heart: individualism and commitment in American life. Berkeley: University of California Press; 1985.
34. Veroff J, Kulka RA, Douvan E. Mental health in America: patterns of help-seeking from 1957 to 1976. New York: Basic Books; 1981.
35. Rieff P. The triumph of the therapeutic: uses of faith after Freud. Wilmington: ISI Books; 2006.
36. Lasch C. The culture of narcissism: American life in an age of diminishing expectations, vol. 1979. New York/London: W.W. Norton; 1979. p. 187.
37. Madsen OJ. The Psychologization of society: on the unfolding of the therapeutic in Norway. Abingdon: Routledge; 2019.
38. Furedi F. Therapy culture: cultivating vulnerability in an uncertain age. London: Routledge; 2004.
39. Conrad P, Bergey M. Medicalization: sociological and anthropological perspectives. In: Wright JD, editor. International encyclopedia of the social & behavioral sciences. 2nd ed. Oxford: Elsevier; 2015. p. 105–9.
40. Horwitz AV, Wakefield JC. The loss of sadness: how psychiatry transformed normal sorrow into depressive disorder. Oxford: Oxford University Press; 2007.
41. Frances A. Saving normal: an insider's revolt against out-of-control psychiatric diagnosis, DSM-5, big pharma, and the medicalization of ordinary life. New York: Morrow; 2013.
42. Watters E. Crazy like us: the globalization of the American psyche. New York: Free Press; 2010.
43. Horwitz AV. PTSD: a short history. Baltimore: Johns Hopkins University Press; 2021.
44. Hacking I. Rewriting the soul: multiple personality and the sciences of memory. Princeton University Press: Princeton; 1995.
45. Kingma E. Naturalist accounts of mental disorders. In: Fulford KWM, Davies M, Gipps RGT, Graham G, Sadler JZ, Stanghellini G, et al., editors. The Oxford handbook of philosphy and psychiatry. Oxford: Oxford University Press; 2013. p. 363–84.
46. Jablensky A. Boundaries of mental disorders. Curr Opin Psychiatry. 2005;18(6):653–8.
47. Slater E. German eugenics in practice. Eugen Rev. 1936;27(4):285–95.
48. Raskin JD. Abnormal psychology: contrasting perspectives. London: Macmillan; 2019.
49. Yakushko O. Eugenics and its evolution in the history of western psychology: a critical archival review. Psychother Politics Int. 2019;17(2):e1495.
50. Cryle P, Stephens E. Normality: a critical genealogy. Chicago: University of Chicago Press; 2017.
51. Rosenhan DL. On being sane in insane places. Science. 1973;179(4070):250–8.
52. Cahalan S. The great pretender: the undercover mission that changed our understanding of madness. Edinburgh: Canongate; 2020.
53. Spitzer RL. More on pseudoscience in science and the case for psychiatric diagnosis: a critique of D. L. Rosenhan's "on being sane in insane places" and "the contextual nature of psychiatric diagnosis". Arch Gen Psychiatry. 1976;33(4):459–70.
54. Klerman GL. The evolution of a scientific nosology. In: Shershow JC, editor. Schizophrenia, science and practice. Cambridge: Harvard University Press; 1978. p. 99–121.

References

55. Kendler KS, Muñoz RA, Murphy G. The development of the Feighner criteria: a historical perspective. Am J Psychiatry. 2010;167(2):134–42.
56. WHO. ICD-11 for mortality and morbidity statistics 2021. Available from: https://icd.who.int/browse11/l-m/en#/http%3a%2f%2fid.who.int%2ficd%2fentity%2f334423054
57. Boorse C. Health as a theoretical concept. Philos Sci. 1977;44(4):542–73.
58. Wakefield JC. The concept of mental disorder: on the boundary between biological facts and social values. Am Psychol. 1992;47(3):373–88.
59. Zachar P. Psychiatric disorders and the imperfect community: a nominalist HDA. In: Faucher L, Forest D, editors. Defining mental disorder: Jerome Wakefield and his critics. Cambridge: MIT Press; 2021. p. 157–75.
60. Lilienfeld S, Marino L. Mental disorder as a Roschian concept: a critique of Wakefield's "harmful dysfunction" analysis. J Abnorm Psychol. 1995;104(3):411–20.
61. Faucher L, Forest D, editors. Defining mental disorder: Jerome Wakefield and his critics. Cambridge: MIT Press; 2021.
62. Wakefield JC. Evolutionary versus prototype analyses of the concept of disorder. J Abnorm Psychol. 1999;108(3):374–99.
63. Biomarkers Definitions Working Group. Biomarkers and surrogate endpoints: preferred definitions and conceptual framework. Clin Pharmacol Ther. 2001;69(3):89–95.
64. Venkatasubramanian G, Keshavan MS. Biomarkers in psychiatry-a critique. Ann Neurosci. 2016;23(1):3–5.
65. Yee CM, Javitt DC, Miller GA. Replacing DSM categorical analyses with dimensional analyses in psychiatry research: the research domain criteria initiative. JAMA Psychiatry. 2015;72(12):1159–60.
66. Plomin R. Blueprint: how DNA makes us who we are. London: Allen Lane; 2018.
67. Bracken P, Thomas P. Postpsychiatry: mental health in a postmodern world. Oxford: Oxford University Press; 2005.
68. Sadler JZ. Conceptual models if normative content in mental disorders. In: Haldipur CV, Knoll JL, et al., editors. Thomas Szaz: an appraisal of his legacy. Oxford: Oxford University Press; 2019. p. 36–52.
69. Rashed MA, Bingham R. Can psychiatry distinguish social deviance from mental disorder? Philosophy Psychiatry Psychology. 2014;21(3):243–55.
70. Prat C. The neuroscience of you: how every brain is different and how to understand yours. New York: Dutton; 2022.
71. Martin MW. From morality to mental health: virtue and vice in a therapeutic culture. Oxford: Oxford University Press; 2006.
72. Legault M, Bourdon J-N, Poirier P. Neurocognitive variety in neurotypical environments: the source of "deficit" in autism. J Behav Brain Sci. 2019;9(06):246–72.
73. Palacios A. The social model in the international convention on the rights of persons with disabilities. Age Hum Rights J. 2015;4:91–110.
74. Richter D, Hertig R, Hoffmann H. Psychiatrische Rehabilitation – von der Stufenleiter zur unterstützten Inklusion. Psychiatr Prax. 2016;43(8):444–9.
75. Keil G, Keuck L, Hauswald R, editors. Vagueness in psychiatry. Oxford: Oxford University Press; 2017.
76. Hyman SE. Psychiatric disorders: grounded in human biology but not natural kinds. Perspect Biol Med. 2021;64(1):6–28.
77. Hofmann B. Vagueness in medicine: on disciplinary indistinctness, fuzzy phenomena, vague concepts, uncertain knowledge, and fact-value-interaction. Axiomathes; 2021.
78. Lilienfeld SO, Treadway MT. Clashing diagnostic approaches: DSM-ICD versus RDoC. Annu Rev Clin Psychol. 2016;12:435–63.
79. Insel T, Cuthbert B, Garvey M, Heinssen R, Pine DS, Quinn K, et al. Research domain criteria (RDoC): toward a new classification framework for research on mental disorders. Am J Psychiatry. 2010;167(7):748–51.

80. Michelini G, Palumbo IM, DeYoung CG, Latzman RD, Kotov R. Linking RDoC and HiTOP: a new interface for advancing psychiatric nosology and neuroscience. Clin Psychol Rev. 2021;86:102025.
81. Kotov R, Krueger RF, Watson D, Achenbach TM, Althoff RR, Bagby RM, et al. The hierarchical taxonomy of psychopathology (HiTOP): a dimensional alternative to traditional nosologies. J Abnorm Psychol. 2017;126(4):454–77.
82. Kotov R, Krueger RF, Watson D, Cicero DC, Conway CC, DeYoung CG, et al. The hierarchical taxonomy of psychopathology (HiTOP): a quantitative nosology based on consensus of evidence. Annu Rev Clin Psychol. 2021;17:83–108.
83. Caspi A, Houts RM, Belsky DW, Goldman-Mellor SJ, Harrington H, Israel S, et al. The p factor: one general psychopathology factor in the structure of psychiatric disorders? Clin Psychol Sci. 2014;2(2):119–37.
84. Caspi A, Moffitt TE. All for one and one for all: mental disorders in one dimension. Am J Psychiatry. 2018;175(9):831–44.
85. Hoff P. On reification of mental illness: historical and conceptual issues from Emil Kraepelin and Eugen Bleuler to DSM-5. In: Kendler KS, Parnas J, editors. Philosophical issues in psychiatry IV: classification of psychiatric illness. Oxford: Oxford University Press; 2017. p. 107–20.
86. Zachar P. Psychiatric disorders: natural kinds made by the world or practical kinds made by us? World Psychiatry. 2015;14(3):288–90.
87. Gewirtz P. On I know it when I see it. Yale Law Journal. 1995;105:1023–47.
88. Andrews D, Toward A. More valid definition of "pornography". J Pop Cult. 2012;45(3):457–77.
89. Szasz TS. The myth of mental illness: foundations of a theory of personal conduct. New York: Harper; 1974.
90. Barrett LF. How emotions are made: the secret life of the brain. London: Pan Books; 2017.

Psychosocial Problems: The Spectrum Model

6.1 Introduction

The conclusion of this book thus far is that coercive measures in psychiatric care can no longer be justified. What follows from this? Although a new legitimisation strategy would be a possible way out, it is not currently apparent in my view, and it would also have to overcome considerable obstacles from a legal perspective and from the point of view of the persons concerned. Another way out could be legal regulation, as proposed by George Szmukler, namely, that people with mental and nonmental illnesses should be treated equally (*fusion law*) to avoid discrimination [1]. According to this proposal, only the determination of incapacity to judge is decisive. However, this creates new difficulties. First, there would have to be a clear demarcation for the presence or absence of mental capacity. However, here, too, one runs into the same methodological problems of dimensional mental characteristics as outlined in the previous chapter [2]. Second, this would not rule out treating people with psychosocial problems against their will. However, it is not only the identification of a "mental disorder" that speaks against coercive measures but also other aspects, such as the predominantly non-existent benefit for the person concerned, which is to be achieved with coercive measures.

Therefore, what might a way out of this legitimisation problem look like? Two essential aspects are the definition of what we call a "mental disorder" and the question of who is authorised to determine a "mental disorder". In this chapter, I suggest that only the person concerned can determine for themselves whether they suffer from a mental disorder and whether they want to seek therapeutic, nontherapeutic or no help at all. Chapter 7 below describes in more detail what human rights-based psychosocial support could look like and how it could differ from previous and current approaches to care. Another aspect is the question of how, and above all, in which setting, to deal with people who do not experience themselves as ill and who pose a risk to themselves or others or who have already committed such acts. This question is addressed in the subsequent Chap. 8.

However, let us first address the question of how and who can determine whether a person is "mentally ill". In the previous chapter, it was concluded that we cannot precisely and, above all, validly define what "mental disorders" are. Nevertheless, human rights violations and coercion in mental health care occur on the grounds of "mental disorders", often against the background of differing perceptions of mental conditions, problems and illnesses between professionals and those affected. This may be related to the individual who shows no "insight" from a clinical perspective or to the question of the existence of mental disorders in general [3]. However, professional insistence on the concept of illness is questionable, as "mental disorders" are not purely biologically or psychologically determined conditions. They cannot be clearly distinguished from one another, nor is the boundary between disorder and non-disorder clearly defined. Nevertheless, these constructs are used both in clinical settings by professionals and laypersons and by members of other fields, such as the legal system or clinical training.

The aim of this chapter is to describe a possible way out of the dilemma that arises from the reality of sociocultural constructs of mental disorders on the one hand and the uncertainties and criticisms of the constructs described in the previous chapter on the other hand. How can we understand psychosocial problems if we take both lines of argumentation seriously? My aim in the following is not to deny the existence of mental disorders but rather to integrate them into a spectrum model that reflects both the disorders and the nonrecognition of this disease concept. My proposal is that we are dealing with mental states that can result in "psychosocial problems" for affected people, and these problems can be described both as a disease and as a non-disease state.

People with psychosocial problems would then have the choice between self-declaration of being ill and self-declaration of not being ill. If such a view were to prevail, the basis for human rights violations in psychiatric care would be removed. No one would be admitted to or treated in a psychiatric ward against his or her will. Psychiatric interventions would be limited to those people who experience themselves as ill and seek medical or therapeutic help on this basis. Exclusive external certification of a "mental disorder" would therefore no longer be permitted.

6.2 From Neurodiversity to Neurocognitive Diversity

In the following sections, I try to outline how one could address the whole issue of mental disorders or illnesses and the rejection of the concept from a social psychiatry perspective. It is therefore also a matter of taking on board the criticism from those affected who do not experience themselves as ill and the criticism from the political and legal system. The latter has been formulated primarily following the United Nations Convention on the Rights of Persons with Disabilities, as I described in the first chapter [4].

It may surprise some readers if I now begin with biological and psychological principles. However, I am convinced of the relevance of biopsychological mechanisms for the development and experience of psychosocial problems. Without

6.2 From Neurodiversity to Neurocognitive Diversity

synaptic connections, no thought or feeling can arise, even if we cannot yet or perhaps never will be able to explain the translation into a subjective experience. There is also no doubt that feelings and thoughts have an effect on other experiences [5]. This is exactly what we experience, even if we do not truly know how it all comes about. As the neuroscientist Antonio Damasio put it in a recently published book, these are "... functional mechanisms that allow us *experience in mind* a process that clearly takes place in the *physical realm of the body*" ([6]: 6).

My starting point is therefore also recent neuroscientific and taxonomic research, which fundamentally assumes the dimensionality of biopsychological facts. Feelings, thoughts and experiences almost always follow a statistical distribution in which boundaries and differences cannot be clearly identified. From the point of view of conventional ICD/DSM psychopathology, comorbidity is one of the central problems. We know that different "disorders", such as anxiety and depression, are highly correlated with each other. As described in the previous chapter, this fact has led to new taxonomic proposals regarding the categorisation of mental disorders in recent years. One prominent proposal is, as mentioned, the "Hierarchical Taxonomy of Psychopathology" (HiTOP) [7, 8] with six psychopathological spectra. Another, even more far-reaching, proposal is the p-factor, i.e. a general psychopathology [9]. If this proposal is followed, it can be assumed that the mental state in the population follows a certain distribution. In this sense, the personality traits of neuroticism, emotional dysregulation, intellectual impairments and thought disorders would be extreme characteristics that are pathologised.

The biopsychological basis is particularly interesting for my approach to psychosocial problems. The p-factor approach sees the foundations both in genetics and in the brain, the central neuropsychological organ. In other words, the population generally has different risks of developing psychological problems in the course of their lives. This risk can also be described using a familiar term as biopsychological vulnerability.

A term often used in this context is "neurodiversity". The terminology originates from the Asperger autism movement and describes the difference and otherness of people who see themselves as "neurodivergent" [10, 11]. Their neurodivergence is therefore based on a biological difference that distinguishes them from people who are considered "neurotypical". Despite their differences, the movement attaches great importance to not being labelled as ill or disabled. Rather, the movement sees itself as a "neurological minority" ([11]: 15) and claims corresponding minority rights.

Different but not ill: this view has been applied to many other phenomena that are labelled disorders in conventional psychopathology, such as ADHD or psychoses. The neurodiversity approach is therefore also seen in the political movement of users/affected people as an approach from which lessons can be learned [12]. At the same time, neurodiversity in clinical psychiatry is seen as a way of complementing the conventional approach to reduce stigmatisation on the one hand and to achieve adjustments in the social environment of those affected on the other hand [13]. In this respect, the neurodiversity approach is quite close to the social model of disability, which does not focus on the person who is disabled but rather on the environment that disables a person who is different from many other people.

As the concept of neurodiversity suggests, the difference from neurotypicals, if the term "neurodiversity" is taken literally, is biologically based. Accordingly, brains are wired differently from those of neurotypicals. Even if the neurodiversity approach explicitly contradicts the label of illness, this suggests a certain proximity to reductionist biological approaches in psychiatry, which answers the following question about the nature of mental disorders as follows: "Brain diseases? Exactly" [14]. This—at least terminologically—reductionism is therefore also met with clear scepticism in parts of the neurodiversity movement [15].

However, other positions seem to have identified a fundamental misunderstanding here. According to them, neurodiversity does not refer exclusively to a biological fact but rather "Neurodiversity is the variation among minds. Every human being differs to some extent from every other human being, with respect to their neurocognitive functioning – how their minds process information and interact with the world. Neurodiversity is the name for this phenomenon" ([16]: 53).

This also corresponds to the state of knowledge in general taxonomic and psychological research, in which biological reductionism is shared less and less. The network approach to psychological syndromes, which has already been cited on various occasions, also counters—in my opinion quite justifiably—"Brain diseases? Not really" [5].

According to this approach, psychological problems are triggered primarily by other psychological phenomena, although these are not independent of biological influences. Rumination promotes sleep disorders, which in turn contribute to a depressed mood, which can then exacerbate sleep disorders and so on.

In line with the impossibility of drawing sharp boundaries between mental disorders and non-disorders described in the previous chapter, taxonomic research also assumes an overwhelming dimensionality of mental phenomena: "(...) people with a mental-disorder diagnosis are not qualitatively different from 'healthy' people. Across the range of human experiences that define mental health and mental illness, people differ in degree, not kind (...)" ([17]: 152). That is, psychological phenomena such as depression are statistically distributed gradually in a population but are not sharply delineated. Some people are more prone to low mood than others are, but low mood as a phenomenon cannot in itself be categorised as "ill" or "disordered".

The same applies to hallucinations, for example. A comprehensive population study in the UK reported a 12-month prevalence of hallucinations of more than 4%. Younger people reported a significantly higher rate than older people did [18]. Delusions, which are conventionally categorised with hallucinations as core symptoms of psychosis, are therefore also not uncommon in the general population. Such studies are already seen as a possible corrective against a clinically distorted view [19], which arises from the fact that clinicians only see people who have significant problems. In contrast, however, there are numerous people with the same experiences who can integrate this perfectly into their everyday lives.

In other words, in addition to neurodiversity, i.e. the diversity of people's biological characteristics, there is also cognitive diversity. The latter means gradually differing experiences and behaviours in the population that cannot be classified as pathological by themselves. However, this does not mean that people cannot suffer from these phenomena. Under certain circumstances, a melancholic state of mind can have such a serious effect that suicide is not only considered but also carried out. Similarly, some voices can be so threatening that the people affected can no longer stand it. However, not being able to bear it is not necessarily pathological, as the discussion about the grief reaction as a possible mental disorder has shown [20]. The loss of a loved one can be an almost unbearable burden and lead to behaviour and experiences that could also be classified as depression. Classification as "disturbed" or "pathological" requires sociocultural factors that contribute to this classification, for example, a diagnostic catalogue that classifies such behaviours and experiences accordingly.

At the end of these considerations, it must therefore be noted that we do not know exactly whether and how to separate two fundamental issues. First, we cannot consistently separate biological and psychological phenomena. Since we cannot say exactly how a thought or a feeling arises from a neuronal impulse, it is advisable to speak of neurocognitive phenomena. Second, as described above, we cannot distinguish between healthy and sick individuals, as neurocognitive phenomena are seen as dimensions. For these reasons, I propose characterising these issues together as "neurocognitive diversity".

6.3 From Neurocognitive Diversity to Sociodiversity

The biological characteristics of a population, such as its genetic or neurobiological disposition, follow a certain distribution. The same applies to mental state, cognitive experience and behaviour. Biology is not determinism, as will be described later. With respect to psychological phenomena, no strict consequences follow from certain biological characteristics. These system levels have their own rules of play and rules of translation; they "irritate" each other by representing environments for the other level [21].

Now, however, there is another level, that of the social. In the sense of causal irritation, social aspects make a not insignificant contribution to what is labelled a mental disorder and what I describe as a psychosocial problem. A comprehensive overview of these issues reveals the following aspects: demographics (including age and gender factors in a population), economics (including social inequality and poverty), the neighbourhood or area in which one lives (including population density and housing development), the wider environment (including wars and conflicts as well as climate change) and sociocultural issues (including social capital and education) [22].

These aspects are key influences on the development and maintenance of psychosocial problems and represent important elements of the social environment. Sociocultural factors in particular are also decisive for the significance of psychosocial problems in a society. The term "looping" has already been used above, which the philosopher Ian Hacking coined to describe the interplay between the sociocultural classification of mental disorders and the psychological experience of the people affected. The following sections focus on these interactions between the mental state and the social environment.

The mutual influence of psychological experience and the social sphere does not take place only in the context of the labelling of sensitivities through diagnoses. First, and this is central to the approach of psychosocial problems, psychological phenomena usually manifest themselves as problems in the social sphere. If a person's depression leads to the point where their ability to work suffers and they are diagnosed as unable to work, they have a social problem. If a person's delusions suggest that they are being poisoned by their partner, then the psychological problem continues to develop into a social problem. If a person's voices command them to attack people physically, then a legal problem looms.

What is important in this context is how tolerant the social environment reacts to experience and behaviour. On a larger scale, social science research has found a clear liberalisation of previously despised, ostracised or even criminalised behaviours in recent decades, especially in Western countries [23]. This liberalisation is also linked to the individualisation already mentioned. Homosexuality, to name one example, is no longer a disease or a criminal offence, as it was 50 years ago in the Western world. Even in the religious and conservative regions of Switzerland, same-sex marriage has now been approved in a referendum. Drug use, at least in the form of cannabis, is also no longer de facto pathologised or criminalised in many countries if it is kept within limits.

Therefore, in many aspects, society has changed into a much less hostile social environment. Of course, and the objections come every time I put forward this thesis, not everything is good and much more could definitely be done in many aspects, and in some areas the opposite is also the case. In psychiatry in particular, we continue to experience a high level of risk aversion, which is reflected, for example, in the increased involvement of child and adult protection authorities in many countries. Numerous behaviours that are labelled as mentally ill, such as psychotic experiences or alcohol addiction, are also still stigmatised. I already mentioned the term "neurotypical" in the previous chapter. This term is used in the context of the neurodiversity movement to characterise the majority in a society. Neurotypicals usually define what is considered a deficit or dysfunction. Nevertheless, there have also been fundamental changes in the way people with disabilities are treated in recent decades. Under the heading of inclusion, attempts are now being made in many areas to make life significantly easier for people with disabilities; here, too, we are experiencing more diversity today than in the past.

The social consequences of mental health problems can be viewed as similarly diverse as neurodiversity or cognitive diversity, namely, as sociodiversity. It can be assumed that identical mental health problems can lead to different social consequences. It depends primarily on the social environment and how well or how badly a person can cope with these difficulties. To give just one example: in a large Western city with a differentiated range of psychosocial services, it is more likely to be able to return to the primary labour market after a mental health crisis as part of a supported employment programme [24]. However, if individuals live in an impoverished rural region of Eastern Europe where such programmes are unknown, the situation is different.

A form of sociodiversity therefore arises when psychological phenomena encounter different social environments. Tolerance, stigmatisation and an implemented psychosocial support service are among the key characteristics that make up sociodiversity in connection with psychosocial problems. Mental health problems not only have psychological consequences but also, especially in the case of severe impairments, social consequences, so it is only logical to categorise them as "psychosocial". In addition to stigmatisation, the social exclusion that many people with psychosocial problems experience should be mentioned here [25]. Social exclusion affects aspects such as income and the labour market, social relationships and intimate relationships or participation in social activities in leisure time. Added to this is—on average—poorer physical health. Many people with pronounced psychosocial problems live in social isolation, feel lonely and experience themselves as cut off from the rest of society [26].

However, another important social circumstance contributes to a further form of sociodiversity. This is the functional differentiation of society into subsystems, as mentioned above. Modern society is not a monolithic entity but rather a complexity of perspectives that can lead to very different views on relevant issues. In recent years, we have witnessed the sometimes drastic differences in perceptions and judgement. The migration crisis, the climate crisis and the COVID-19 pandemic have led not only to public controversy but also to physical attacks on people. Rarely have we seen modern society as polarised and emotionalised in connection with these issues.

The pandemic, like previous epidemics [27], has made it clear that even in relation to diseases, there is no automatic mechanism for arriving at a common view. This means that scientific issues are also sociocultural issues such as religion, child education or transport policy. Just because science has reached a far-reaching near-consensus, such as on the climate issue or in the fight against the pandemic, this does not mean that everyone else agrees and will follow the proposals.

I believe that this problem can be used to demonstrate quite plausibly how modern society works, namely, functional differentiation. An essential realisation of the sociology of modern societies is that there can no longer be any authority or truth, such as premodern religion. Truths and other certainties that were binding for all people have disappeared with the transition to modern society. Modern society, on the other hand, is characterised by the fact that various subsystems, such as politics, law, science and economics, observe each other without one of the subsystems being able to assume superiority. When politicians claimed during the pandemic that they followed science entirely, this was only true as long as there was no fear of massive losses in the next elections [28]. Social subsystems follow their own rules and can at best be irritated but not controlled from outside [29].

Of course, the scientific system cannot do without publishing its research results as "true"—research results that would be declared "false" from the outset would have no chance of being published. However, it is not absolute truths that are proclaimed there but only scientific truths, i.e. observations of a subsystem of society.

Science "...cannot claim an exceptional position for itself and see itself in the role of an external observer who describes reality (however imperfectly) as it is" ([30]: 667). Nevertheless, if it attempts to do so, as can sometimes be observed, it is quickly convicted of naivety by political, economic or media realities. A differentiated society produces context-dependent observations, and the scientific context is only one of many. Modern society is polycontextual.

From a sociological perspective, it is therefore not surprising that other subsystems, such as the legal system or the political system, judge "mental illness" differently from the scientific mainstream. Reference has already been made on several occasions in this book to the United Nations and its suborganisations, which in recent years have adopted a completely different view of psychiatric interventions such as coercive measures. In their view, these are not therapeutic interventions but rather come closer to human rights violations or even torture [31].

In a polycontextural society, it is not possible for everyone to determine who is right in this matter. From the perspective of most clinicians, coercive measures are interventions that enable therapies, if not therapeutic in themselves. From the perspective of the legal system, which refers to the UN CRPD, for example, this looks different in some respects. What applies to coercive measures also applies to the issue of "mental illness". In the broader context of the UN CRPD, the term "psychosocial disability" is therefore used rather than illness. In legal research, this is seen as a paradigm shift in favour of a social model of disability and, moreover, towards full equality and inclusion of affected persons [32].

6.4 Psychosocial Problems in a Socio-diverse Context

The terminology of "psychosocial disability" just quoted goes back to the not inconsiderable influence of the *World Network of Users and Survivors of Psychiatry*, *WNUSP*, on the development of the UN CRPD. According to WNUSP, "psychosocial disability" is the preferred term for people who define themselves as: "users or consumers of mental health services; survivors of psychiatry; people who experience mood swings, fear, voices or visions; mad; people experiencing mental health problems, issues or crises" [33].

This is therefore about the self-declaration of people who experience themselves as limited in the context of a mental health problem. This is associated with a viewpoint that conspicuously does not speak of "illness" or "mental disorder" but also does not exclude the use of mental health care. Non-consensus perspectives on mental health issues have been increasingly endorsed within the service user community [34]. Likewise, this self-definition does not exclude the possibility that the people it refers to are experiencing crises or health problems. In other words, these are people who experience themselves as different and/or have experienced mental health crises and reject the label of illness or disorder.

The fact that the rejection of the label or even the doubts are not unjustified is confirmed by the neuroscientific research already cited several times, even if the WNUSP user movement makes no reference to this. To repeat a central thesis from the previous chapter, we do not truly know what a mental disorder is. Nevertheless, many people are completely convinced of the existence of mental disorders and illnesses. The willingness to seek treatment is increasing significantly, as almost all relevant empirical indicators suggest. The increase in the prescription and probably also the use of psychotropic medication is particularly remarkable. In all OECD countries, i.e. primarily Western and developed countries, the consumption of antidepressants roughly doubled between 2000 and 2017 [35]. In Switzerland, the consumption of antidepressants rose by almost 50 percent between 2007 and 2017, and the use of psychiatric or psychotherapeutic practices rose by approximately 20 percent [36].

A certain socio-diversity in dealing with psychosocial problems can also be recognised here. Certainly, the majority of the population interprets psychosocial problems as illnesses. Otherwise, the utilisation of corresponding services would not be very high and would not continue to increase. In addition, presumably many service users experience an improvement in their problems. In this respect, the concept of illness is certainly plausible. For many affected users of institutionalised forms of care, however, the situation is sometimes different. They have always viewed the concept of illness with a certain degree of scepticism, and this scepticism does not seem implausible either. Their experiences may not have been so favourable, and institutional psychiatry in particular has not always been very welcoming and empathetic to the concerns of many users.

6.5 Psychosocial Problems: The Spectrum Model

From a scientific perspective that takes into account basic neuroscientific research as well as epistemological, philosophical and sociological aspects, neither the concept of mental illness nor the rejection of the concept can be denied a certain degree of comprehensibility. Similarly, none of the positions can be prioritised. There are neither empirical nor epistemological reasons for prioritising the affirmative or the negative model [37]. What a "mental illness" or a "mental disorder" means is historically and culturally contingent. This means that the terminology and associated concepts could have developed quite differently. The historical contingency can be plausibly illustrated by describing the considerable change in psychiatric illness concepts on the one hand and the self-image of people with certain mental phenomena on the other hand.

The philosopher and historian of science, Ian Hacking, has addressed these questions in several works. One of his starting points was the first description of autism in 1943 by the Austrian-American psychiatrist Leo Kanner. Before 1943, no one associated the concept of autism with children. The scientific and epistemological question now is, did autism even exist before 1943? In retrospect, this is almost an idle question. However, viewed prospectively, for example, from the year 1930, it looks different. The same question could be asked: do mental illnesses already exist today that we do not even know about yet? There is no valid answer to this question.

Ian Hacking solved this problem empirically [38]. It is, he says, absurd to assume that autism did not exist before 1943. However, before 1950, and actually before the mid-1970s, people did not experience themselves in this way. The people affected did not interact with their families, their social contacts or the support system as autistic people did. However, this has changed since the 2000s. People with corresponding psychological phenomena then perceived themselves as such and, when problems arose, sought help under the label of "autism". The background of this development is the "looping" phenomenon already mentioned in the previous chapter: self-classifications are influenced by medical classifications and findings. This makes it clear that both the identification of an "illness" and the self-perception associated with it are historically and culturally contingent. The entire process of classification and self-classification is dependent on numerous unpredictable and, to a certain extent, random social events and developments. Conversely, there is therefore no compelling need to define mental illness exclusively in the conventional medical sense or to reject this concept completely.

How does the assessment of being ill or not ill relate to other characteristics and influencing factors? Figure 6.1 outlines the spectrum model of psychosocial problems. The starting point of the spectrum model is biological and psychological diversity. Against the background of the current state of research, it is now possible to describe more precisely the levels at which the biological factors, the psychological factors and the social or sociocultural factors make themselves felt. Figure 6.1 shows that all of these influences are understood as spectra. In this context, it is important to emphasise the predominantly non-deterministic relationships between the different levels. In biological research, various genotype-phenotype processes are currently assumed to produce variability in a population. There is a discussion of stochastic (i.e. random) relationships, as well as non-deterministic and, in certain

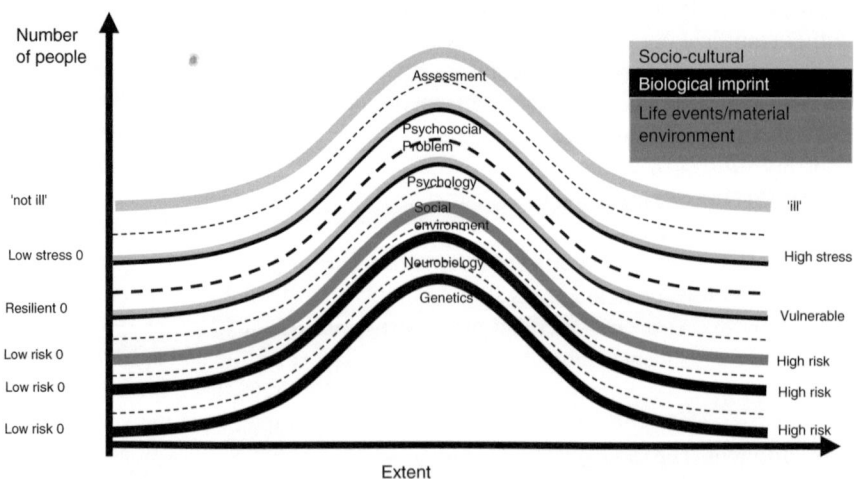

Fig. 6.1 Spectrum model

cases, deterministic associations [39]. As only a two-dimensional representation of the relationships is possible here, the broken lines are intended to indicate this fact.

At the genetic level, there is a diversity that leads to corresponding risks of developing certain biological or psychological characteristics [40]. A certain genetic profile therefore increases the risk of becoming more vulnerable or resilient, more likely to hear voices (or not) or to have a more depressive world view (or not). The same also applies to neurobiological variability [41] or, using the terminology used here, neurobiological diversity. Moreover, certain characteristics can increase or decrease the risk for the abovementioned (and many other) characteristics.

The psychological level is somewhat more complicated. Here too, psychological diversity in terms of low to high stress is also assumed. As will be explained shortly, variation is the norm. This is where biological and sociocultural factors collide, as indicated in Fig. 6.1. There is now extensive evidence of sociocultural influences on psychological phenomena such as emotions [42, 43], which differ across cultures [44]. This interplay between biology and socioculture also has an impact on psychological vulnerability or resilience [45].

In connection with the sociodiversity of modern societies, reference has already been made to the different social characteristics of people with psychosocial problems, such as income or social networks. The distribution of or changes in these characteristics are correlated with psychosocial problems, which should be assessed in the same way as genetic or neurobiological correlations [46].

The slightly thicker dashed line in Fig. 6.1 separates the psychological phenomena and the biological, psychological and social influences acting on them from the psychosocial problems and their assessment. Psychosocial problems are thought of as a combination of biological, psychological and social characteristics. These problems, in turn, lie on a spectrum that describes the stress.

6.6 From a Psychological Phenomenon to a Psychosocial Problem

However, how is it that psychological phenomena or conditions become psychosocial problems? To answer this question, we need to go back a little and refer to current neuroscience. One of the most promising theories at present is the *active inference* approach [47, 48]. This approach is part of a research programme in *computational psych*iatry [49], which assumes that the central function of the human brain is prediction. According to current research, the human brain does not process information but rather constructs it. This means that the flow of information does not go from the outside to the inside, from the environment to the brain, as we intuitively assume. Contrary to human intuition, it is exactly the other way around, from the brain actively into the respective environment [50].

Active inference goes back to the mathematical theories of Thomas Bayes, an eighteenth-century English theologian who became known less for his theology than for his work on statistics and probability theory and whose theory enjoys considerable popularity today in statistics [51] and in the philosophy of science [52].

Bayes' problem was—to put it very simply—the question of how likely an event is to occur if we take certain prior information into account when predicting it.

The relationships among previous states, assumptions and expectations as well as subsequent perceptions are also central to active inference. At its core, it is about minimising uncertainty and surprises. This approach is compatible with more recent theories of consciousness, which were described in Chap. 5. Perception, according to one of the basic assumptions there, arises from predictions about the environment and the subjective information that I filter out of my environment. We therefore have no direct access to our environment but construct our perception by constantly comparing our expectations with sensory information. Ultimately, according to various theories from psychology [53] and philosophy [54], we "hallucinate" incessantly. The crucial question here is how well our hallucinations fit in with what we perceive as our environment, i.e. how well we can control our hallucinations.

As one of the few neuroscientific approaches, active inference establishes a direct connection to the social environment; not least for this reason, the theory is promising in my view. Problems arise when our hallucinations become uncontrollable in the sense that assumptions and expectations do not correspond with information from the environment. In other words, problems arise when we are unable to adapt our assumptions appropriately to the environment or are unable to adapt our environment to our assumptions. Dealing with uncertainty in the social environment is an initial situation that can lead to anxious or depressive states, for example. Interestingly, our own body is also one of the relevant environments. The perception of one's own body and its functions (interoception) plays a central role in the development of emotional states and problematic situations [42, 55].

This means that active inference can also be linked to neurocognitive diversity [43]. Our constructed perceptions and emotions lie—as should have become clear by now—on a spectrum. This spectrum includes "neurotypical" constructs that are shared by the majority but also less typical constructs that are perceived as divergent. In the context of the diagnosis of anorexia nervosa (AN), for example, this approach concludes "...that AN patients have inferred a model of their basic homeostatic state that deviates dramatically from the expectations defining the typical human phenotype" ([56]: 223).

Contrary to what is assumed in conventional psychiatric research, the heterogeneity of phenomena is not a nuisance that we recognise after the usual assumption of essences or *natural kinds*. Lisa Feldmann Barrett, one of the leading emotion researchers, stated in this regard that "(w)e need to accept variability as the norm and not as a nuisance that we explain away once it has been identified" ([42]: 16). Attempts to combine these approaches from mathematical psychiatry with the voice hearing movement [57] go even further by positively supporting the normalisation of voice hearing. In both approaches, for example, it is assumed that voice hearing is more likely to be present in the context of uncertainty.

Neurocognitive diversity is therefore the norm and, to a certain extent, normality. However, the normality of diversity does not prevent conditions from becoming problems in certain situations and psychosocial constellations. Psychosocial problems arise when the constructs of our perception, i.e. our mental states, have negative consequences. These consequences occur mainly when certain variations of the state's conflict with the social environments in which they perceive themselves or when the effects are perceived by other people: "No kind of mind is inherently better or worse than any other. Some variations are just more tailored to their environment" ([58]: 109).

6.7 Mentally Ill or Not: The Assessment Spectrum

Conversely, this means that there are variations in mental states that do not fit well into their respective environments. These include, for example, suffering from the personal or social condition (as is often the case with depressive states). However, there can also be social consequences (e.g. if the social environment no longer accepts the condition or behaviour). The problems can then take different forms. They can be short-term and crisis-like, they can take on a longer duration and they can also take the form of a disability in the sense of the UN CRPD, i.e. a psychosocial disability. However, all these forms of psychosocial problems do not necessarily imply that they have to be regarded as "illness" or "disorder".

However, it is of course not impossible to see a psychosocial problem as a "disorder". The Dutch philosopher Sanneke de Haan, after also supporting many of the arguments put forward here in her book on *Enactive Psychiatry*, nevertheless argued in favour of the term "disorder" over "differences". Her reasoning: "Because normalisation can fail to do justice to the experiences of those who suffer from psychiatric disorders…" ([59]: 205). And de Haan is of course right that we must provide those who suffer from certain problems with the support they need. However, she is not right when she necessarily classifies this as a disorder. Moreover, by her own admission, de Haan also runs into the problem of where to draw the line between disorder and non-disorder.

In my view, these difficulties and supposed contradictions can be resolved relatively easily. The assessment of a psychosocial problem in terms of "ill" or "not ill" also lies on a spectrum. In other words, whether a psychosocial problem should be considered an illness or a disorder can and is in fact assessed differently. The assessment is the responsibility of the people affected. They should be able to decide in general or on a case-by-case basis whether the psychosocial problem they are experiencing should be regarded as an illness or not. However, this also means that an exclusively external assessment of a psychological phenomenon or a psychosocial problem as pathological is not permissible. The assessment of the person affected by these phenomena or problems is decisive.

Therefore, from a social psychiatry perspective in particular, the people affected by psychosocial problems must be given the freedom to choose how they themselves assess their condition. It is therefore a matter of preference for their concept of the problem and their self-concept of how they want to behave towards the problem. A key aspect in this context is whether they want to seek help or support.

In the case of a disease/disorder position, it is likely that those affected see biological, psychological or social factors as relevant. According to experience and individual subjective assessments, these can be genetic in the biological sense, for example, if other family members are or were also affected by the same problem. However, affected persons can also claim intrapsychic conflict in the psychological sense, such as dependency versus autonomy. Alternatively, they may consider a social event to be particularly relevant, for example, a psychological trauma or a stressful life event such as the loss of a loved one.

However, if people with psychosocial problems "decide" against the disease/disorder label, this could also give rise to different explanatory patterns. To name just a few of the possibilities, this would initially be the description as "I am different, but not ill" in the sense of the neurodiversity approach. However, it could also be that the person themselves does not experience what is seen as a problem from the outside as problematic at all. This can occur, for example, in connection with the use of psychotropic substances if people from the environment attribute this as excessive or even pathological, while the person in question perceives their lifestyle as not accepted. It is well-known that the perception of others and self-perception can differ drastically in connection with psychological phenomena. Finally, as experience in supporting people in outpatient residential settings shows, many people with psychosocial problems are happy to make use of support without experiencing themselves as ill. It is possible to suffer from certain social constellations or psychological phenomena without immediately seeing this as being "ill".

As surprising or even absurd, as the preference model may sound with respect to disease status, it is already accepted in certain parts of mental health care. An important example in this context is "hearing voices". When I started working in mental health nursing in the 1980s, "auditory hallucinations" had an exclusively negative connotation in the sense of a psychotic symptom that had to be treated with neuroleptics. This has changed in various ways in recent decades owing to the commitment of those affected and of some clinicians. Without wanting to underestimate the stressful or even threatening nature of the voices, many studies have demonstrated how a different assessment of the voices is possible [60]. Hearing voices can thus be reinterpreted from a symptom to a neutral psychological phenomenon or experience. Voices can have a subjective meaning or biographical significance for some, for example, in connection with traumas experienced or other detrimental problems in their lives [61]. Hearing voices even has positive aspects for some people affected by them, insofar as they can be part of their individual identity. This finding also has implications for supportive approaches and the concept of psychosis. Among the supportive approaches, there are both self-help approaches, such as the voice-hearing movement [62], and dialogue-based approaches, which can involve professionals [63]. If voice hearing is viewed as a neutral phenomenon, psychosis can also be reconceptualised as a phenomenon by de-medicalising and de-psychiatrising it [64].

Another psychotic phenomenon, delusion, has also recently been scientifically described as more than just a negative or dysfunctional symptom. As is easy to imagine, ideas of grandeur can have positive connotations. People with delusions also describe the feeling of suddenly seeing and understanding many things more clearly and coherently. These phenomena certainly have a threatening effect on

6.7 Mentally Ill or Not: The Assessment Spectrum

many of those affected, but there are also reports of neutral to indeed positive effects from delusions [65].

The same applies to the so-called Asperger syndrome within the autism spectrum. Many people with Asperger traits do not experience themselves as deficient but as neurodivergent in the sense of being different from so-called neurotypicals [66]. This diversity does not necessarily have to be viewed negatively, as many neurodivergents are highly functional in many social circumstances. A special pride in being different is emphasised by the *Mad Pride* movement [67, 68]. In analogy to queer lifestyles and the "body positivity" of people with a higher body weight, "mad positivity" is emphasised here, i.e. the positive experiences that madness can bring.

In addition, as hard as it may be to accept, the "Pro Ana" or "Pro Mia" movements of women with altered eating behaviours, clinically characterised as anorexia or bulimia, are heading in the same direction. For many young women (and some young men), altered eating behaviour—as life-threatening and health-threatening as it can be—is a lifestyle that meets their needs and preferences [69]. "Pro Ana" is an expression of neurocognitive and social diversity, where perceptions about one's own and other bodies are often fuelled by cultural influences that are now primarily communicated through social media.

What is considered sick or healthy in the psychiatric field, or even what is considered functional or dysfunctional, is a question of perspective, and the dominant perspective is usually determined from the point of view of the majority in a society. Incidentally, this is no different when dealing with assumptions about "mental illness" than when dealing with ethnic or racial stereotypes, as was already established at the end of the 1970s [70]. Even then, the author of this publication concluded, "These stereotypes will persist until the actual relations between groups, including their relative power, begin to change" ([70]: 221). Currently, the power of institutional psychiatry is somewhat eroded, with peers and other people affected by psychosocial problems being found not only in the support of users but also in teaching, research and even in the management of psychiatric services.

The fact that these are stereotypes projected by the majority onto the minority of neurodivergents can shed light on a reversal of perspectives. The autism researcher and activist Damian Milton coined the term "double empathy problem" in this context [71]. The starting point of his analysis is the so-called "Theory of Mind" problem associated with autistic people [72]. This was based, first, on the observation that autistic people find it difficult to communicate and, second, on the conviction that autistic people have difficulties adequately understanding what is happening in other people's minds. In other words, they would have empathy problems and difficulty developing an adequate theory of other people's mental states.

The "double empathy problem" approach now states that autistic people do indeed have difficulties cognitively empathising with other people. However, this also applies in the other direction: neurotypical people have problems cognitively empathising with autistic people. The "deficit" or "dysfunction" is therefore not solely on the part of the autistic person. The mutual empathy problem has been confirmed by recent empirical research, which shows that autistic people can communicate with each other more easily than is the case with non-autistic people [73].

and that neurotypical people find people with autism significantly less likeable than non-autistic people [74]. There are obviously misunderstandings on both sides; however, as usual, the deficits tend to be attributed to the minority.

6.8 Conclusion: Disease Definition as a Perspective Construct

These examples should clarify how much the self-characterisation of ill or not ill can depend on the respective perspective, the subjective experience, the extent of suffering from the phenomenon or the wider sociocultural context and the respective social environment. Neurocognitive diversity is therefore generally also associated with sociodiversity. Ultimately, therefore, it is a choice in the sense of a preference as to whether one's own mental state is regarded as a pathology. Certainly, suffering from the phenomenon is more likely to be associated with the characterisation of illness, but this does not necessarily have to be the case. A person can suffer from certain phenomena and circumstances but may perceive or decide for themselves that they do not want to consider it an illness.

The different backgrounds of psychosocial problems naturally suggest that different preferences regarding support and/or treatment are associated with the description of the problems. If a problem is labelled "ill", the person may be more willing to seek medical treatment and possibly more willing to accept medication. These aspects are described in more detail in a subsequent chapter. If the possibly distressing phenomena are not considered in the context of illness, the picture is predictably contradictory. However, even within the two positions of "ill" or "not ill", there will not be complete agreement on the acceptance or rejection of medical treatments.

All of these findings suggest that not only the individual concept of experiencing psychological phenomena should be understood as a preferable approach but also the measures that can contribute to an improvement in psychological distress, if it is subjectively present. The following chapter attempts to describe what I see as the necessary shift towards human rights-based psychosocial support.

References

1. Szmukler G. Men in white coats: treatment under coercion. Oxford: Oxford University Press; 2018. 01 Dec 2017
2. Richter D. Coercive measures in psychiatry can hardly be justified in principle any longer—ethico-legal requirements versus empirical research data and conceptual issues. J Psychiatr Ment Health Nurs. 2025;32(2):461–6.
3. Dixon J, Richter D. Contemporary public perceptions of psychiatry: some problems for mental health professions. Soc Theory Health. 2018;16(4):326–41.
4. United Nations. UN convention on the rights of persons with disabilities 2006.. Available from: https://www.un.org/development/desa/disabilities/convention-on-the-rights-of-persons-with-disabilities/convention-on-the-rights-of-persons-with-disabilities-2.html.

5. Borsboom D, Cramer AOJ, Kalis A. Brain disorders? Not really: why network structures block reductionism in psychopathology research. Behav Brain Sci. 2018;42:e2.
6. Damasio A. Feeling & knowing: making minds conscious, vol. 12. New York: Pantheon Books; 2021. p. 65.
7. Kotov R, Krueger RF, Watson D, Achenbach TM, Althoff RR, Bagby RM, et al. The hierarchical taxonomy of psychopathology (HiTOP): a dimensional alternative to traditional nosologies. J Abnorm Psychol. 2017;126(4):454–77.
8. Kotov R, Krueger RF, Watson D, Cicero DC, Conway CC, DeYoung CG, et al. The hierarchical taxonomy of psychopathology (HiTOP): a quantitative nosology based on consensus of evidence. Annu Rev Clin Psychol. 2021;17:83–108.
9. Caspi A, Moffitt TE. All for one and one for all: mental disorders in one dimension. Am J Psychiatry. 2018;175(9):831–44.
10. Silberman S. Neurotribes: the legacy of autism and how to think smarter about people who think differently. London: Allen and Unwin; 2015.
11. Singer J. NeuroDiversity: the birth of an idea. n.p: Amazon; 2017.
12. Graby S. Neurodiversity: bridging the gap between disabled people's movement and the mental health survivors' movement? In: Spandler H, Anderson J, Sapey B, editors. Madness, distress and the politics of disablement. Bristop: Policy Press; 2015. p. 231–43.
13. Sonuga-Barke E, Thapar A. The neurodiversity concept: is it helpful for clinicians and scientists? Lancet Psychiatry. 2021;8(7):559–61.
14. Insel TR, Cuthbert BN. Medicine. Brain disorders? Precisely. Science. 2015;348(6234):499–500.
15. Russel G. Critiques of the neurodiversity movement. In: Kapp S, editor. Autistic community and the neurodiversity movement. Singapore: Palgrave Macmillan; 2020. p. 287–303.
16. Walker N. Neuroqueer heresies: notes on the neurodiversity paradigm, autistic empowerment, and postnormal possibilities. Fort Worth: Autonomous Books; 2021.
17. Conway CC, Krueger RF. Rethinking the diagnosis of mental disorders: data-driven psychological dimensions, not categories, as a framework for mental-health research, treatment, and training. Curr Dir Psychol Sci. 2021;30(2):151–8.
18. Yates K, Lång U, Peters EM, Wigman JTW, McNicholas F, Cannon M, et al. Hallucinations in the general population across the adult lifespan: prevalence and psychopathologic significance. Br J Psychiatry. 2021;1-7:652.
19. Harper DJ. Realising the potential of general population research to reconceptualise the study of "delusions": from normalising "psychosis" to defamiliarising "normality". Theory Psychol. 2021;31(6):887. https://doi.org/10.1177/09593543211000429.
20. Horwitz AV, Wakefield JC. The loss of sadness: how psychiatry transformed normal sorrow into depressive disorder. Oxford: Oxford UP; 2007.
21. Richter D. Psychisches System und soziale Umwelt: Soziologie psychischer Störungen in der Ära der Biowissenschaften. Bonn: Psychiatrie-Verlag; 2003.
22. Lund C, Brooke-Sumner C, Baingana F, Baron EC, Breuer E, Chandra P, et al. Social determinants of mental disorders and the sustainable development goals: a systematic review of reviews. Lancet Psychiatry. 2018;5(4):357–69.
23. Inglehart RF. Cultural evolution: people's motivations are changing, and reshaping the world. Cambridge: Cambridge University Press; 2018.
24. Richter D, Hunziker M, Hoffmann H. Supported Employment im Routinebetrieb: Evaluation des Berner Job Coach Placement-Programms 2005–2016. Psychiatr Prax. 2019;46(06):338–41.
25. Richter D, Hoffmann H. Social exclusion of people with severe mental illness in Switzerland: results from the Swiss health survey. Epidemiol Psychiatr Sci. 2019;28(4):427–35.
26. Cogan NA, MacIntyre G, Stewart A, Tofts A, Quinn N, Johnston G, et al. "The biggest barrier is to inclusion itself": the experience of citizenship for adults with mental health problems. J Ment Health. 2021;30(3):358–65.
27. Richter D. War der Coronavirus-Lockdown notwendig? Versuch einer wissenschaftlichen Antwort. Bielefeld: Transcript; 2021.

28. Richter D, Zuercher S. The epidemic failure cycle hypothesis: towards understanding the global community's recent failures in responding to an epidemic. J Infect Public Health. 2021;14:1614.
29. Luhmann N. Die Gesellschaft der Gesellschaft. Frankfurt/M: Suhrkamp; 1997.
30. Luhmann N. Die Wissenschaft der Gesellschaft. Frankfurt/M: Suhrkamp; 1990.
31. UN General Assembly. Report of the special rapporteur on torture and other cruel, inhuman or degrading treatment or punishment, Juan E Méndez 2013.. Contract No.: A/HRC/22/53.
32. Doyle GS. The right to liberty of persons with psychosocial disabilities at the United Nations: a tale of two interpretations. Int J Law Psychiatry. 2019;66:101497.
33. WNUSP. Psychosocial disability: World Network of Users and Survivors of Psychiatry; 2008. Available from: https://www.ohchr.org/Documents/Issues/CulturalRights/CulturalHeritage/Submissions/13.2.WNUSP-Appendix2.docx.
34. Speyer H, Ustrup M. Embracing dissensus in lived experience research: the power of conflicting experiential knowledge. Lancet Psychiatry. 2025;12(4):310–6.
35. OECD. Health at a Glance – 2019 Health Indicators 2019. Available from: https://doi.org/10.1787/888934018146.
36. Schuler D, Tuch A, Peter C. Psychische Gesundheit in der Schweiz. Neuchâtel: Schweizerisches Gesundheitsobservatorium; 2020. Contract No.: 15/2020
37. Richter D, Dixon J. Models of mental health problems: a quasi-systematic review of theoretical approaches. J Ment Health. 2023;32(2):396–406.
38. Hacking I. Kinds of people: moving targets. Proc Br Acad. 2007;151:285–318.
39. Hiesinger PR, Hassan BA. The evolution of variability and robustness in neural development. Trends Neurosci. 2018;41(9):577–86.
40. Moreno-De-Luca D, Martin CL. All for one and one for all: heterogeneity of genetic etiologies in neurodevelopmental psychiatric disorders. Curr Opin Genet Dev. 2021;68:71–8.
41. Bethlehem RAI, Seidlitz J, White SR, Vogel JW, Anderson KM, Adamson C, et al. Brain charts for the human lifespan. Nature. 2022;604(7906):525–33.
42. Barrett LF. The theory of constructed emotion: an active inference account of interoception and categorization. Soc Cogn Affect Neurosci. 2016;12(1):1–23.
43. Barrett LF. How emotions are made: the secret life of the brain. London: Pan Books; 2017.
44. Mesquita B. Between us: how cultures create emotions. New York: Norton; 2022.
45. Shaffer C, Westlin C, Quigley KS, Whitfield-Gabrieli S, Barrett LF. Allostasis, action, and affect in depression: insights from the theory of constructed emotion. Annu Rev Clin Psychol. 2022;18(1):553–80.
46. Thomson RM, Igelström E, Purba AK, Shimonovich M, Thomson H, McCartney G, et al. How do income changes impact on mental health and wellbeing for working-age adults? A systematic review and meta-analysis. Lancet Public Health. 2022;7(6):e515–e28.
47. Friston K, FitzGerald T, Rigoli F, Schwartenbeck P, Pezzulo G. Active inference: a process theory. Neural Comput. 2017;29(1):1–49.
48. Parr T, Pezzulo G, Friston KJ. Active inference: the free energy principle in mind, brain, and behavior. Cambridge, MA: MIT Press; 2022.
49. Friston KJ, Stephan KE, Montague R, Dolan RJ. Computational psychiatry: the brain as a phantastic organ. Lancet Psychiatry. 2014;1(2):148–58.
50. Buzsáki G. The brain from inside out. Oxford: Oxford UP; 2019.
51. Lee PM. Bayesian statistics: an introduction. 4th ed. Chichester: Wiley; 2012.
52. Sprenger J, Hartmann S. Bayesian philosophy of science. Oxford: Oxford UP; 2019.
53. Seth AK. Being you: a new science of consciousness. London: Faber; 2021.
54. Clark A. Surfing uncertainty: prediction, action and the embodied mind. Oxford: Oxford UP; 2016.
55. Clark JE, Watson S, Friston KJ. What is mood? A computational perspective. Psychol Med. 2018;48(14):2277–84.
56. Gadsby S, Hohwy J. Why use predictive processing to explain psychopathology? The case of *Anorexia Nervosa*. In: Mendonca D, Curado M, Gouveia SS, editors. The philosophy and science of predictive processing. London: Bloomsbury; 2021. p. 209–26.

57. Powers AR III, Bien C, Corlett PR. Aligning computational psychiatry with the hearing voices movement: hearing their voices. JAMA Psychiatry. 2018;75(6):640–1.
58. Barrett LF. Seven and a half lessons about the brain. London: Picador; 2020.
59. de Haan S. Enactive psychiatry. Cambridge: Cambridge UP; 2020.
60. Woods A, Romme M, McCarthy-Jones S, Escher S, Dillon J. Special edition: voices in a positive light. Psychosis. 2013;5(3):213–5.
61. McCarthy-Jones S, Castro Romero M, McCarthy-Jones R, Dillon J, Cooper-Rompato C, Kieran K, et al. Hearing the unheard: an interdisciplinary, mixed methodology study of women's experiences of hearing voices (auditory verbal hallucinations). Front Psych. 2015;6:181.
62. Longden E, Read J, Dillon J. Assessing the impact and effectiveness of hearing voices network self-help groups. Community Ment Health J. 2018;54(2):184–8.
63. Burr C, Schnackenberg JK, Weidner F. Talk-based approaches to support people who are distressed by their experience of hearing voices: a scoping review. Front Psychiatry. 2022;13:983999.
64. Higgs RN. Reconceptualizing psychosis: the hearing voices movement and social approaches to health. Health Hum Rights. 2020;22(1):133–44.
65. Ritunnano R, Kleinman J, Whyte Oshodi D, Michail M, Nelson B, Humpston CS, et al. Subjective experience and meaning of delusions in psychosis: a systematic review and qualitative evidence synthesis. Lancet Psychiatry. 2022;9(6):458–76.
66. Chapman R, Carel H. Neurodiversity, epistemic injustice, and the good human life. J Soc Philos. 2022;53:614.
67. Hoffman GA. Public mental health without the health? Challenges and contributions from the mad pride and neurodiversity paradigms. In: Cratsley K, Radden J, editors. Developments in neuroethics and bioethics. 2: Academic; 2019. p. 289–326.
68. Rashed MA. Madness and the demand for recognition: a philosophical inquiry into identity and mental health activism. Oxford: Oxford UP; 2019.
69. Roberts Strife S, Rickard K. The conceptualization of anorexia: the pro-ana perspective. Affilia. 2011;26(2):213–7.
70. Townsend JM. Stereotypes of mental illness: a comparison with ethnic stereotypes. Cult Med Psychiatry. 1979;3(3):205–29.
71. Milton DEM. On the ontological status of autism: the 'double empathy problem'. Disabil Soc. 2012;27(6):883–7.
72. Baron-Cohen S. Mindblindness: an essay on autism and theory of mind. Cambridge, MA: MIT Press; 1997.
73. Mitchell P, Sheppard E, Cassidy S. Autism and the double empathy problem: implications for development and mental health. Br J Dev Psychol. 2021;39(1):1–18.
74. Alkhaldi RS, Sheppard E, Burdett E, Mitchell P. Do neurotypical people like or dislike autistic people? Autism Adulthood. 2021;3(3):275–9.

Human Rights-Based Psychosocial Support

7.1 Introduction

The conclusion from the previous chapter was that people with psychosocial problems should decide for themselves whether they consider themselves to be ill or not. An exclusively external assessment, the validity of which cannot be guaranteed, should therefore no longer be permitted. This step would remove a key building block for the legitimisation of coercive psychiatric measures, as these are often based solely on the opinion of a specialist with regard to the definition of illness.

Psychosocial support in accordance with individual preferences prevents restrictions and thus the violation of personal rights. In the following, however, the focus will be not only on prevention but also on the question of how human rights-based support can be imagined in a positive sense. What distinguishes human rights-based support from current and previous forms of care? What elements of support can be considered and in what form? The Quality Rights initiative of the World Health Organisation (WHO) has already proposed several aspects in this direction: respect for legal capacity, care without coercion, user participation, social inclusion, and recovery [1]. This direction will be developed more systematically in the following sections.

7.2 Human Rights Development in Mental Health Care

The human rights orientation and associated psychosocial support lie in meeting the preferences of service users and other affected persons. In a nutshell, it is about preference-based psychosocial support. Clinicians in the mental health care context should primarily follow what service users want. An essential aspect of the following remarks is the outline of ideal human rights-based support for the future, which, however, is already visible in parts today and has already been implemented to some extent.

Where the future is concerned, however, the present and the past must also be considered, as described in Chap. 3. In this context, I propose dividing mental health care since its beginning in the nineteenth century into three major phases in which the rights of the people affected by care were dealt with differently. The first phase, which lasted in Europe until around the 1960s/1970s, largely disregarded human rights. The human rights and civil liberties of people committed to asylums or institutions were generally ignored. The people concerned were mostly there against their will, and many had to spend years and sometimes decades in the institution. The medical procedure was generally determined by medical specialists who were able to rely on their professional and, where available, academic authority.

This was followed in the 1980s by a phase that is still dominant today. This phase can be characterised by the fact that human rights are acknowledged but can be restricted for medical reasons. Person-centredness and evidence-based approaches play decisive roles in this phase. The approach was to organise primarily medical psychiatry in the assumed interests of the users on the basis of scientific evidence of the forms of therapy.

Certain changes in terms of human rights are now to be seen, at least in outline. The next phase of psychosocial support with a distinct social psychiatry flavour should be human rights-based support. Its aim is to fully safeguard the fundamental rights and freedoms of the people receiving psychosocial support. Instead of "person-centred", the term "person driven" is now used [2].

7.3 What Support Preferences Do People with Psychosocial Problems Have?

During the human rights-ignoring phase of mental health care described above, there can be little talk of the preferences of the people affected. This should begin to change with the phase in which human rights were acknowledged but could nevertheless be considerably restricted for medical reasons—or more precisely, can still be restricted. There is now extensive research on treatment and support preferences in medicine in general [3, 4]. Similar studies are also available for psychiatry [5]. These findings reveal the following broader picture. First, pharmacological interventions are less popular with users than counselling or psychotherapy [6, 7]. Second, institution-based services are less favoured than outpatient or outreach services in their own home [8, 9].

As is usually the case with such survey studies that report group-related results, it must be taken into account that preferences are very heterogeneous. Not all people with psychosocial problems have the same ideas about how they want to be supported and what is important to them. The specific goals that people have presumably depend on numerous factors, such as whether and how ill they experience themselves or what goals they generally pursue in their lives. An interesting study from the United States identified three major groups of people with psychosis in this regard: people who want to achieve something in their lives, people who tend to seek stability and people who are health-oriented [10]. The specific goals to be achieved also vary depending on the basic orientation. For example, a full-time job is expected to be sought predominantly by people who are more achievement-oriented. This group also tends to want to live in their own home and earn as much money as possible. What they have in common with the health-oriented group is that they do not want to experience voices or other unusual things. In contrast, this was less important for the stability-oriented group. This group also had less clear preferences for a high income, possibly because they had less pleasant experiences in the labour market.

These findings suggest that the life goals and support preferences of people with psychosocial problems are highly individualised and should be treated as such. This means that clinicians and other professionals should not assume conformist ideas ("people with X certainly want Y") but should instead—as with all people—enquire in each individual case and support the decision in question accordingly. This is particularly emphasised here because the ideas about appropriate goals and approaches very often differ among professionals, users and other stakeholders, such as relatives [11].

Furthermore, it is important for me to emphasise that the characterisation of today's mental health care as a purely neoliberal commercial venture for the pharmaceutical industry and the "psy-professions" (e.g. [12, 13]) misses the core of the problem. In the course of the book, I described the social constructivist background to "illness" and cited the sometimes-low effectiveness of therapies. Moreover, it is of course true that entire industries and professions live from medicalisation and psychologisation and therefore benefit from it. However, the call for a de-medicalisation of psychosocial problems and the characterisation of, for example, antidepressants as a myth [14] leads to an epistemic injustice towards those who, with the help of professional support and pharmacology, can lead to a stable and liveable life. If it helps, benefits and does not harm these people from their perspective, what should speak against it?

Medicalisation and psychologisation contribute significantly to coping with the sometimes difficult and aversive conditions of life in modern society. It is certainly not wrong to emphasise "… that the concept of an illness is not required to understand the aetiology of a large number of problems currently considered to represent some form of illness…" ([15]: 11). From this statement, the authors conclude that psychopathology should be depathologised. However, the same applies here as before: If people with psychosocial problems interpret them as "illness", as happens millions of times, and this helps them to understand their problems and to deal with them, what should speak against it? A medicalised and psychologised perspective on personal problems is the dominant view in the Global North today. A medicalised and psychologised perspective therefore has the same right to exist as the rejection of this perspective. From a social psychiatry and mental health nursing perspective in particular, it should be possible for the perspectives to exist and stand side by side on an equal footing. If this is not possible, the epistemic injustice that we criticise from an exclusively biomedical perspective would be promoted.

7.4 From Shared Decision-Making to Supported Decision-Making

On several occasions, the United Nations Convention on the Rights of Persons with Disabilities (UN CRPD) has created new foundations for the understanding of disabilities and impairments as well as for psychiatric care. This applies in particular in the context of decision-making by professionals and affected persons or users. The background here is the legal capacity of people with disabilities, which can generally be restricted by national or regional legal systems, often in a significant way. In contrast, Article 12 of the UN CRPD emphasises the goals "...that persons with disabilities have the right to recognition everywhere as persons before the law" and that measures should be taken "... to provide access by persons with disabilities to the support they may require in exercising their legal capacity" [16]. In other words, people with disabilities should be able to make their own decisions about their legal affairs, and professionals should support them so that they can actually do so. This is essentially the legal view, which could lead to the abolition of legal representatives such as guardians or legal carers [17] if they are appointed against the will of the person concerned.

However, this principle can, of course, be applied not only in connection with legally relevant decisions. As in the field of physical medicine, where this approach is sometimes called "informed decision-making" [18], this approach can and should also be the norm in psychosocial care—up to and including decisions on measures that could involve coercion [19]. From a human rights perspective, which favours decisions on the basis of will and preference, it can generally be assumed that people with psychosocial problems can decide for themselves what is the right choice for them in terms of support, care and treatment, even if they need assistance to come their right choice. This is what 'supported decision-making' means.

In some countries, physical care has already gone further than psychiatric care. The British *Royal College of Surgeons* (RCS) issued standards back in 2016 that declare supported decision-making to be a principle [20]. The background to this was an obstetric case in which a patient was not informed of certain risks and her child was born with birth defects [21]. The UK Supreme Court subsequently ruled that it was not permissible to provide information based on clinical judgement but that all such information should be disclosed for the purposes of informed choice. Interestingly, the standards required by the RCS also include the option of no treatment. According to the document, if patients are capable of judgement, it must be accepted that they do not receive treatment, even if this is contrary to clinical judgement and medical ethics.

In the relevant psychiatric research literature, institutional or communicative approaches such as "Open Dialogue", peer support or Soteria houses and wards are among the implementations of supported decision-making [22]. This is hardly surprising given that the same approaches are regarded by the World Health Organisation (WHO) as exemplary for the implementation of a human rights-based approach in line with the UN CRPD [1]. As will become clear in a moment, these approaches are not considered particularly effective in terms of the evidence-based psychiatry practised today. Apart from the fact that this may be due to methodological circumstances, the question remains as to whether scientific evidence should always take precedence over the preference of the user in psychosocial support [23]. In supported decision-making, there is, as is easy to imagine, a certain risk from the clinician's point of view that the beneficiaries will decide against the scientific evidence.

In this context, however, it is important to remember various aspects that are relevant here. First, it can be assumed that many users are strongly oriented towards biomedicine and are prepared to accept scientific evidence as decisive in terms of decision-making [24]. Second, however, it should be remembered that the evidence for the effectiveness of psychiatric treatment is not particularly strong, as I show in Chap. 4. In this respect, the argument that one must follow evidence-based psychiatry is not particularly convincing. Third, it should be remembered that the methods of evidence-based medicine (EBM) today have moved quite far away from how they were developed in the 1990s. Even back then, the danger was recognised that EBM would be applied in a cookbook-like manner, with decisions being made solely on the basis of studies [25]. However, EBM, in the sense of its original approach, was based on a high value of clinical expertise, which should be incorporated into the medical decision-making process. Furthermore, the entire decision-making process should be characterised by "... the more thoughtful identification and compassionate use of individual patients' predicaments, rights, and preferences in making clinical decisions about their care" ([26]: 71). Supported decision-making is obviously not thus far removed from EBM in the initial sense.

7.5 Supported Decision-Making: Preference over Evidence

Evidence-based support or preference-based support is therefore one of the crucial questions in connection with the decision-making of people with psychosocial problems. As can be expected, my answer is that preferences are the most important factor, and scientific evidence comes into play when service users have a support or treatment preference that has been scientifically verified. What does that mean in concrete terms? The principles of Soteria treatment, as implemented in the 1970s and 1980s in the United States and then later in Europe, included acute psychiatric care without neuroleptics or later with a relatively low antipsychotic pharmacological dose [27]. However, as is easy to understand, this low-dose therapy is less successful in achieving the treatment goal of preventing a first or second psychotic relapse [28].

Now the conventional conclusion is as follows: especially at the beginning of psychotic development, treatment should not be carried out at a low dosage. On the other hand, from my perspective, the question would be how relevant the risk of a psychotic relapse is from the perspective of the person affected, especially against the background of the not inconsiderable side effects of a higher dose. If relapse prevention is not a high priority, this should also be reflected in the dose of antipsychotics—if medication is accepted at all. However, if relapse prevention is the top priority, the person should be informed about the effects and side effects of the dose in an evidence-based manner to make the decision criteria more transparent and facilitate the decision. This is where preferences come into play again. A higher antipsychotic dose is associated with more side effects [29]. If this is accepted in view of the prioritisation of relapse prevention, the evidence-based form of therapy and dose of medication would ultimately come into play here. If the side effects are not acceptable, alternative non-drug support strategies should be discussed.

It is perfectly possible to formalise the procedure outlined above via a generic algorithm. Figure 7.1 describes the decision paths. From the point of view of the person concerned, there is a psychosocial problem (e.g. psychotic experience) for which a preferred solution is sought (in this example, the solution could be called Open Dialogue procedure or medication). As the name suggests, the Open Dialogue process is an outreach, systemic and communication-based process that attempts to reach decisions in the event of a severe mental health crisis with the involvement of all parties [30]. Therefore, evidence may be available for the preferred solution (medication) or not (Open Dialogue). If the person opts for the solution without evidence, this is nevertheless the procedure, and Open Dialogue is used. If they decide in favour of evidence, all information regarding effects and side effects should be disclosed. The next step is to assess whether the evidence is acceptable,

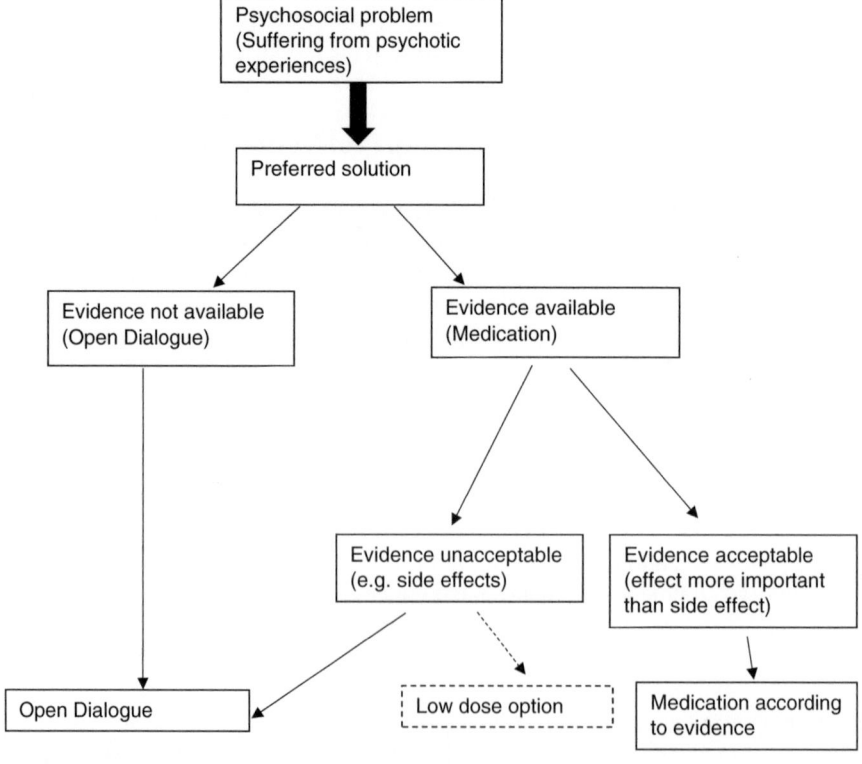

Fig. 7.1 Preference versus evidence—decision algorithm

i.e. whether the effect of the drug is considered sufficient, even in view of the side effects. If this is not the case, non-drug solutions should be considered, or a lower dose should be prescribed. Otherwise, the medication is administered in accordance with the evidence.

In other words, evidence-based decisions are always relevant in the care of people with psychosocial problems if the goals favoured by the users have been evaluated with regard to their achievement via appropriate research methodology. This approach is a reversal of the usual approach in many parts of mental health care, but it is compatible with the initial evidence-based medicine of the 1990s.

According to current research, a good therapeutic alliance between a professional and a person with a psychosocial problem is crucial for the effectiveness and sustainable implementation of supported decision-making [31, 32]. Trust is therefore key. Affected persons must be able to trust that the professional will provide all relevant information and communicate this in an appropriate and, above all, comprehensible form. It must also be possible to trust that the preferences will ultimately be implemented in the measures that are deemed necessary.

A fundamental problem in the therapeutic alliance between clinicians and people with psychosocial problems, which can only be overcome with trust, is the undoubted power asymmetry that exists. Professionals usually have more and better information at their disposal, and they generally also have the ability to achieve their goals through communication. This may be the reason why peer counselling is generally held in high regard by those affected or those who use it. In contrast to peers, professionals are perceived as more goal-oriented, whereas peers are seen as more process-oriented [33]. Presumably, the preferences of users can be discussed and weighed more openly and appropriately in discussions with peers than is the case with conventionally trained staff.

7.6 Human Rights-Based Psychosocial Support: Person-Centred and Preference-Based

The history of human rights in psychiatry can be divided into three phases, as described above: disregarding human rights (phase 1), acknowledging human rights (phase 2) and human rights as the basis of support (phase 3). The right-hand column of Table 7.1 lists what I consider to be the essential aspects of human rights-respecting psychosocial support. These aspects are supplemented by what I consider to be essential in the earlier phases 1 and 2. In such a concise list, nuances and certain variations are naturally lost, especially as the phase of disregard for human rights spans approximately two centuries.

To respect human rights, the *focus of support* must no longer be on institutions, as in the past (phase 1), or on person-centredness, as at present (phase 2), but on person-driven management (phase 3). As correct and important as person-centredness was, its shortcomings became clear, for example, in that psychiatric coercion could certainly be justified as a person-centred measure [34].

Table 7.1 Human rights phases in psychiatry

	Disregarding human rights (Phase 1)	Acknowledging human rights (Phase 2)	Human rights as a basis (Phase 3)
Focus	Institution-centred	Person-centred	Person-driven
Decision criterion	Eminence (medical-scientific authority)	Scientific evidence	Preference of the person
Ethical approach	Social norms, interest of the family	Well-being of the person concerned	Will and preference of the person concerned
Legal basis	Mainly involuntary	Involuntary hospitalisation and treatment in certain circumstances; formal voluntariness, but widespread informal and administrative coercion	Exclusively voluntary
Legal capacity	Mostly refused	Restricted under certain circumstances	Extensively granted
Coercion	Predominantly forced placement and treatment	Forced placement and other measures not the rule, but happen often	No coercion in care; normality principle; quarantine in case of ongoing risk to others
Place of care/support	Hospital/institution	Hospital and community	According to preference
Supply/support model	Institutional psychiatry	Social and community psychiatry	Psychosocial support according to preference (also exclusively medical treatment)
Disease model	Psychodynamic, biomedical	Biopsychosocial	Psychosocial problems—plurality of models
Health model	None	Absence of symptoms, later quality of life	Psychosocial health—individual priorities, including recovery
Importance of symptoms	Suppressed	Treated	Relevance and handling depending on preference
Importance of the diagnosis	Broad diagnostic groups, prognostic function	Central feature of the treatment and the organisation of the treatment	According to preference and disease model

7.6 Human Rights-Based Psychosocial Support: Person-Centred and Preference-Based

	Accommodation	Treatment/care	Support according to preference (treatment/care/coaching/peer support)
Professional approach			
Objective	Monitoring the person	Symptom management	Individual goals (according to preference)
Main intervention	Compulsion/physical therapies/medication	Medication/psychotherapy for special indications	According to preference
Medication	Often by force/without consent	Prescription, possibly against the will	Professionally supported self-determined intake/non-intake
Professions in the support system	Dominance of the medical profession	Multi-professional team under medical management	Multi-professional team without professional group dominance; inclusion of service users as peer support; ideally inclusion of peers in the management of programmes
Needs/requirements	Physical requirements, if any	"Objective" psychosocial needs/requirements (plus satisfaction and quality of life)	Subjective psychosocial and/or physical needs
Deficits/strengths	Deficit-orientation	Balance of deficits and resources	Predominantly resource-orientated
Risk orientation	Harm/risk avoidance	Risk minimisation/risk management	Dealing constructively with risks (positive risk-taking)
Balance of power	In favour of the professionals	Intended but not realised balance	According to preference
Social goal	Social exclusion	Social integration	Social inclusion
Rehabilitation	None (living and working in the institution)	Stepladder/linear continuum	Supported inclusion
Research	Users as involuntary objects of research	Mental disorder including the user's perspective (e.g. satisfaction and quality of life)	Active involvement of users in research planning and implementation
Professional training/university teaching	Service users as exposed objects	Service users as objects of clinical training	Service users as teachers

Person-centredness does not exclude coercion. With person-driven control, this is the sole responsibility of the person affected by any action.

***

This means *that the decision criterion* for what should happen in the support is the preference of the person concerned. In earlier times, this was the eminence in the person of the medical or scientific authority [35] and, later, the scientific evidence. In essence, there must be a change from evidence to preference.

***

The importance of the preference of the person concerned is also prominent in the central *ethical approach* of human rights-based phase 3. Whereas in phase 1, it was the social norms and the interests of the family, this changed in phase 2 to the supposed benefit of the person concerned, whereas now it is the will and preference of the person, as is also expressed in the UN CRPD.

***

The *legal basis* for support, care and treatment must therefore be exclusively voluntary. It must no longer be determined by formal, informal or administrative coercion. In the institution-centred phase, which disregards human rights, people were predominantly treated involuntarily, whereas in the present day, this is predominantly done formally on a voluntary basis. Nevertheless, many people are affected by measures taken against their will, not to mention widespread informal and administrative coercion.

***

This means that the *legal capacity* of the person concerned should no longer be restricted in the future, as is still the case today in almost all legal systems around the world. Legal capacity must be fully granted, as required by Article 12 of the UN CRPD [36].

***

Coercion was widely used during the human rights abuse phase. This is less the case today. The use of coercion, in any form, is fundamentally inadmissible in support of human rights. Exceptions to this are self-binding directives in which people have determined what should happen if, in their judgement, they can no longer make appropriate decisions [37]. Such agreements are also called "Ulysses clauses". As a reminder, in Homer's "Odyssey", the protagonist had himself tied to the ship because he feared that he would not be able to resist the sirens' enticing song. The next chapter explains what principles and options a modern society must have to be able to deal appropriately with people who pose risks to themselves or to others. It also describes the dilemma situations that can arise.

***

In the past, *the place of care and support* was more or less exclusively the asylum/hospital or the institution, as it was called at the time. In the context of deinstitutionalisation and dehospitalisation during psychiatric reforms, services

7.6 Human Rights-Based Psychosocial Support: Person-Centred and Preference-Based

increasingly shifted to the community, and pure institutional psychiatry became the community psychiatry that is predominantly found today [38]. However, hospitals still have a central function in many regions, as some services are only available there. Human rights-based support would stipulate that the place of care is up to the service user's preference.

***

In the context of support that respects human rights, the *type of support* is up to the preferences of the person concerned, too. This does not preclude people from seeking conventional pharmacological and/or psychotherapeutic treatment, nor does it preclude hospital treatment; the decisive factor is the person's preference.

***

In terms of *disease models*, there has been development from the biomedical and psychoanalytical concepts of earlier decades towards a—at least envisaged—biopsychosocial model [39]. However, the latter has been controversial for some time [40], and the question is to what extent it has been applied at all [41]. Preference-oriented support relies on diverse models of psychosocial problems, especially as there is no obvious argument in favour of one particular model over others [42]. According to the spectrum model of psychosocial problems described in the previous chapter, preference is also decisive here.

***

This also corresponds to the concept of psychosocial *health*. This concept first developed in the person-centred phase, which took human rights into account, in the direction of the absence of symptoms, as typically recorded in the context of standardised psychopathological assessments. Only around the turn of the last century were further aspects such as quality of life surveyed [43]. Psychosocial health in the context of support that respects human rights is not only an individual concept that can also include the absence of symptoms but also aspects such as personal recovery, which is about finding meaning despite or perhaps even because of psychosocial problems [44].

***

The concepts of illness and health also correspond to the different ways of dealing with the phenomena called *symptoms* in the respective phases. Whereas in the era of disregard for human rights, the primary aim was to suppress the phenomena without treatments being available, in recent decades, they have become the actual goal of treatment. The predominant pharmacological approaches are aimed at assessing psychopathological symptoms. The relevance of these phenomena, whether they are even assessed as "symptoms" of an "illness", is, in turn, a matter for the affected persons themselves in a support system that respects human rights. The frequently cited example of hearing voices and dealing with them can show the path that needs to be taken.

***

The different approaches to *diagnoses* also correspond to the concepts of illness and health. In the early days of classification systems, these systems were rather broadly based and had primarily prognostic functions [45]. The diagnosis subsequently became the central feature of treatment, organisation and reimbursement. Special wards, in which people with the same diagnoses are treated, have been increasingly implemented in recent decades. However, many of these wards have already been abandoned in favour of the so-called track system [46]. The track system claims to offer more flexibility and autonomy. In a support system that is person-centred and preference-based, this should be determined entirely by the people concerned. Diagnoses lose their significance if the individual disease model does not go hand in hand with them. However, diagnoses can be very valuable in providing affected people with a better understanding of their psychosocial problems. This means that for many users, a diagnosis can be meaningful and useful; for others, it can mean stigma and discrimination [47].

***

Now to the support itself: The general *professional approach in* the early phase of psychiatry consisted primarily of the accommodation and segregation of the affected person from their social environment, and above all, in separation from the family ([48]: 89ff.). For a long time, there were no forms of therapy available that were even minimally effective. This changed only in the second half of the twentieth century, where treatment and (nursing) care were the central professional approaches in the phase that took human rights into account. However, this also implied treatment against the person's will. Therefore, support that respects human rights requires modified and additional support options that can be chosen according to preferences, such as coaching, peer support and communicative interventions such as Open Dialogue. In particular, the inclusion of peers as people also affected by psychosocial problems can be an essential step toward building trust in non-medicalised support systems, for example, in dealing with suicidal tendencies [49].

***

The predominant *objective* in the human rights disregarding phase was monitoring. This was replaced by the treatment goal of symptom management. Psychopathology was the focus of treatment in the human rights-acknowledging phase. Individual goals, which can also lie beyond phenomena and symptoms, should be the focus of support in the future. These can be not only aspects of everyday professional or social life but also non-pharmacological forms of coping that make it easier to address certain phenomena [50].

***

The main *interventions* in the early phase were often coercion as an end in itself to monitor and control people, followed by physical interventions such as lobotomy, a psychosurgical measure that is now regarded as one of the greatest mistakes in medicine [51]. The second phase, which took human rights into account, initially continued to work with biological interventions, even without the consent of the patients concerned. Furthermore, pharmacological therapy was the primary

7.6 Human Rights-Based Psychosocial Support: Person-Centred and Preference-Based

measure, although individual indications were and are treated psychotherapeutically. However, to respect human rights by taking into account the individual preferences of the people receiving support, further options are required in the proposed next phase, which have already been mentioned above in connection with professional approaches.

***

Relevant *forms of medication* were not available in psychiatry until the 1960s [52]. As described, these were often administered by formal and informal coercion without the actual consent of those affected. In the human rights acknowledging phase, this was duly prescribed, but forced medication has not disappeared to this day. In Switzerland, more than 3% of inpatients recently received forced medication [53]. It goes without saying that this should no longer happen if human rights are respected. Rather, the aim is for people receiving support to learn to use medication in a self-determined way. If medication is helpful, it can be an important component of psychosocial stabilisation. If they are experienced as unhelpful or even detrimental to health, they need to be handled differently, which may include professionally supervised discontinuation of medication [54].

***

In the era of psychiatry, which disregarded human rights, the medical profession developed as the dominant *profession*. The second major professional group was initially the untrained "lunatic attendant", from which mental health nursing developed. In the current phase, we find the so-called multi-professional team, which—with certain exceptions—is still led by the medical profession for historical and legal reasons. To do justice to the preferences of the people to be supported, a multi-professional team without a dominant professional group but with the involvement of peers is required as a minimum. Ideally, peers will also be involved in the management of support services in a further step [55]. However, these roles also require a certain amount of experience.

***

In the first centuries of psychiatric care, the focus was not on mental *needs and requirements* but, at best, on physical needs. Even these were often not dealt with in the best interests of the people being cared for, given the brutal coercive measures and later interventions and medication administered against their will. In connection with the concept of person-centredness, it became clear in the phase in which human rights were taken into account how much person-centredness was based on "objective" indicators of need and not on the subjective needs of the people concerned. This then changed to some extent with the consideration of quality of life and user satisfaction in the 1990s [56]. In human rights-based support, however, subjective psychological, social and physical needs should be at the centre of care. The dilemmas caused by this, for example, in social law matters, are discussed in the following chapter.

***

The history of psychiatry is also a history of *deficit orientation*; even certain sexual orientations were characterised as mental deficits [57]. We are currently experiencing a certain tendency towards resource orientation in the phase in which human rights are taken into account [58]. Overall, however, we can only assume a balance between deficit orientation and resource orientation. This should continue to change towards a primary resource orientation if human rights are not only taken into account but also respected. Even if it is perhaps not politically opportune at present to refer to deficits and problem situations, this cannot be dispensed with. Without deficits and problems, no support would be utilised. The difference from current practices is the significance of resources and deficits, which should change in favour of resources.

***

As the French sociologist Robert Castel noted, the history of psychiatry has seen a change in the way people categorised as mentally ill have dealt with the harms and *risks* they appeared to pose. This change took place from the perception of harm to risk [59]. As already indicated on various occasions, many people with psychosis were initially generally regarded as dangerous to the public. Later, in the human rights-acknowledging phase 2, risk assessment and risk management were and still are at the centre of attention; I described this in connection with the legitimisation of coercion in Chap. 2. In a human rights-based phase, this should have changed in the direction of a positive approach to risk (*positive risk taking*). In the future, it will not be a question of avoiding risks but rather of consciously taking risks under certain circumstances and learning from any problems and mistakes. At present, many employees in mental health services still find this quite difficult, as risk avoidance0 is still a widespread attitude [60, 61]. Certainly, this also has to do with possible legal consequences if damage occurs. The legal system is not geared towards a positive approach to risk.

***

For many centuries, the relationship between clinicians and service users or people affected by psychiatry was an asymmetrical *balance of power* in favour of the staff. In fact, this is still the case today. Although concepts such as the joint/shared decision-making described above have aimed to achieve a balance of power [62], this approach has rarely been implemented in routine care [63]. However, shared decision-making does not go far enough in terms of the UN CRPD. This calls for supported decision-making [64], which changes the power asymmetry in favour of the user. It is also important to take preferences into account here. Not all users want to make self-determined decisions; some also agree with professionally determined decisions about their treatment and support.

***

The social goal of psychiatry in the phase of human rights abuse was social exclusion. Not all but many people had to spend several years to decades in institutions, separated from their social environment against their will. In the phase that respected human rights, the goal of social integration developed [65]. The human rights goal of social inclusion [66], which essentially means adapting the social environment to the needs of the person to be supported, is already recognizable to some extent in today's practice. Within Supported Employment programs, for example, we see such adaptations of the working environment to people's needs.

***

The models of *psychiatric rehabilitation* correspond with social goals. Initially, virtually no rehabilitation was aimed at living and working in the hospital or institution, and occupational therapy was seen as something that was intended to support "healing" [67]. The rehabilitation goal of integration was to be achieved in the subsequent phase via the so-called step ladder or linear continuum principle [68]. As with medical rehabilitation in general, there was a conviction that increasing stress and strain would enable the person concerned to regain the necessary competences by adapting to the social environment. Today, we know that most users do not achieve their social integration goals by climbing the ladder. Furthermore, inclusion does not mean adapting to the environment but adapting the environment to the person's needs in the sense of supported inclusion [69]. Again, Supported Employment is a good example of this adaptation.

***

Chapter 3 has already described how service users or people affected by psychiatry generally became involuntary objects of psychiatric *research*; this was common during the human rights abuse phase. The issue not only affected psychiatry but also disenfranchisement was greater here than in other areas of medicine, as most people affected by research were involuntarily accommodated and treated. This was not to formally change psychiatry until the 1964 "Declaration of Helsinki" by the World Medical Association [70]. Today, the requirement of informed consent for study participants applies to all medical research. In the human rights phase, increasing emphasis was also placed on the perspective of users, for example, through surveys on satisfaction and quality of life. Research that respects human rights also requires the active participation of users/affected persons in research projects, which are ideally also developed and managed by them [71].

***

A similar story can be observed for the role of users/affected persons in *professional training and university teaching*. Here too, for decades, users/affected persons were also objects that were presented to students and probably also to the wider public in lecture theatres [72]. This practice changed over time, but I can still remember so-called tribunal ward rounds, in which service users sat opposite several clinicians seated in a semi-circle. Such ward rounds were used in the presence of the users for training purposes, among other goals. However, to make the perspectives of users/affected people clear in the context of human rights-based support, active and ideally leading involvement of affected people is needed, as in previous research [73]. The motto should also apply to training: "Nothing about us without us."

7.7 Conclusions: Building Blocks of Person-Centred Support

In my opinion, the contrast with previous and current practices in psychiatric care has made it possible to highlight the steps towards human rights that are already visible today but also those that need to be taken. In many places, the simple solution is that the preferences of the users and those affected should decide what to do and what not to do.

However, the implementation of such preference-based support faces many hurdles. Numerous legal, ethical and practical problems and dilemmas must be recognised and dealt with along the way. The penultimate chapter addresses the specific difficulties and possible solutions.

References

1. WHO. Guidance on community mental health services: promoting person-centred and rights-based approaches. Geneva: World Health Organisation; 2021.
2. SAMHSA. SAMHSA's working definition of recovery. Substance Abuse and Mental Health Services Administration; 2012.
3. Yu T, Enkh-Amgalan N, Zorigt G. Methods to perform systematic reviews of patient preferences: a literature survey. BMC Med Res Methodol. 2017;17(1):166.
4. Ho M, Saha A, McCleary KK, Levitan B, Christopher S, Zandlo K, et al. A framework for incorporating patient preferences regarding benefits and risks into regulatory assessment of medical technologies. Value Health. 2016;19(6):746–50.
5. Larsen A, Tele A, Kumar M. Mental health service preferences of patients and providers: a scoping review of conjoint analysis and discrete choice experiments from global public health literature over the last 20 years (1999–2019). BMC Health Serv Res. 2021;21(1):589.
6. McHugh RK, Whitton SW, Peckham AD, Welge JA, Otto MW. Patient preference for psychological vs pharmacologic treatment of psychiatric disorders: a meta-analytic review. J Clin Psychiatry. 2013;74(6):595–602.
7. Winter SE, Barber JP. Should treatment for depression be based more on patient preference? Patient Prefer Adherence. 2013;7:1047–57.
8. Richter D, Hoffmann H. Preference for independent housing of persons with mental disorders: systematic review and meta-analysis. Admin Pol Ment Health. 2017;44(6):817–23.
9. Farrelly S, Brown G, Rose D, Doherty E, Henderson RC, Birchwood M, et al. What service users with psychotic disorders want in a mental health crisis or relapse: thematic analysis of joint crisis plans. Soc Psychiatry Psychiatr Epidemiol. 2014;49(10):1609–17.
10. Zipursky RB, Cunningham CE, Stewart B, Rimas H, Cole E, Vaz SM. Characterizing outcome preferences in patients with psychotic disorders: a discrete choice conjoint experiment. Schizophr Res. 2017;185:107–13.
11. Lasalvia A, Boggian I, Bonetto C, Saggioro V, Piccione G, Zanoni C, et al. Multiple perspectives on mental health outcome: needs for care and service satisfaction assessed by staff, patients and family members. Soc Psychiatry Psychiatr Epidemiol. 2012;47(7):1035–45.
12. Esposito L, Perez FM. Neoliberalism and the commodification of mental health. Humanit Soc. 2014;38(4):414–42.
13. Tseris E. Biomedicine, neoliberalism and the pharmaceuticalisation of society. In: Cohen BMZ, editor. Routledge international handbook of critical mental health. Abingdon: Routledge; 2018. p. 169–76.
14. Moncrieff J. The myth of the antidepressant: an historical analysis. In: Rapley M, Moncrieff J, Dillon J, editors. De-medicalizing misery: psychiatry, psychology and the human condition. Basingstole: Palgrave Macmillan; 2011. p. 174–88.

References

15. Wasserman T, Wasserman LD. Depathologizing psychopathology: the neuroscience of mental illness and its treatment. Cham: Springer; 2016.
16. United Nations. UN convention on the rights of persons with disabilities 2006. Available from: https://www.un.org/development/desa/disabilities/convention-on-the-rights-of-persons-with-disabilities/convention-on-the-rights-of-persons-with-disabilities-2.html.
17. Gooding P. Supported decision-making: a rights-based disability concept and its implications for mental health law. Psychiatry Psychol Law. 2013;20(3):431–51.
18. van der Heide I, Uiters E, Jantine Schuit A, Rademakers J, Fransen M. Health literacy and informed decision making regarding colorectal cancer screening: a systematic review. Eur J Pub Health. 2015;25(4):575–82.
19. Newton-Howes G, Kininmonth L, Gordon S. Substituted decision making and coercion: the socially accepted problem in psychiatric practice and a CRPD-based response to them. Int J Mental Health Capacity Law. 2020;26:4–12.
20. RCS. Consent: Supported Decision-Making: Royal of College of Surgeons; 2016. Available from: https://www.rcseng.ac.uk/standards-and-research/standards-and-guidance/good-practice-guides/consent/.
21. Chan SW, Tulloch E, Cooper ES, Smith A, Wojcik W, Norman JE. Montgomery and informed consent: where are we now? Br Med J. 2017;357:j2224.
22. Penzenstadler L, Molodynski A, Khazaal Y. Supported decision making for people with mental health disorders in clinical practice: a systematic review. Int J Psychiatry Clin Pract. 2020;24(1):3–9.
23. Gupta M. Is evidence-based psychiatry ethical? Oxford: Oxford UP; 2014.
24. Knight F, Kokanović R, Ridge D, Brophy L, Hill N, Johnston-Ataata K, et al. Supported decision-making: the expectations held by people with experience of mental illness. Qual Health Res. 2018;28(6):1002–15.
25. Sackett DL. Evidence-based medicine. Semin Perinatol. 1997;21(1):3–5.
26. Sackett DL, Rosenberg WMC, Gray JAM, Haynes RB, Richardson WS. Evidence based medicine: what it is and what it isn't. BMJ. 1996;312(7023):71–2.
27. Calton T, Ferriter M, Huband N, Spandler H. A systematic review of the Soteria paradigm for the treatment of people diagnosed with schizophrenia. Schizophr Bull. 2008;34(1):181–92.
28. Taipale H, Tanskanen A, Correll CU, Tiihonen J. Real-world effectiveness of antipsychotic doses for relapse prevention in patients with first-episode schizophrenia in Finland: a nationwide, register-based cohort study. Lancet Psychiatry. 2022;9:271.
29. Leucht S, Crippa A, Siafis S, Patel MX, Orsini N, Davis JM. Dose-response meta-analysis of antipsychotic drugs for acute schizophrenia. Am J Psychiatry. 2020;177(4):342–53.
30. Seikkula J, Olson ME. The open dialogue approach to acute psychosis: its poetics and micropolitics. Fam Process. 2003;42(3):403–18.
31. Dixon J, Donnelly S, Campbell J, Laing J. Safeguarding people living with dementia: how social workers can use supported decision-making strategies to support the human rights of individuals during adult safeguarding enquiries. Br J Soc Work. 2021;52:1307.
32. Webb P, Davidson G, Edge R, Falls D, Keenan F, Kelly B, et al. Key components of supporting and assessing decision making ability. Int J Law Psychiatry. 2020;72:101613.
33. Bochicchio L, Stefancic A, McTavish C, Tuda D, Cabassa LJ. "Being there" vs "being direct:" perspectives of persons with serious mental illness on receiving support with physical health from peer and non-peer providers. Adm Policy Ment Health Ment Health Serv Res. 2021;48(3):539–50.
34. Rudnick A. Commentary: can seclusion and restraint be person-centered? Isr J Psychiatry Relat Sci. 2013;50(1):11–2.
35. Bhandari M, Zlowodzki M, Cole PA. From eminence-based practice to evidence-based practice: a paradigm shift. Minn Med. 2004;87(4):51–4.
36. Arstein-Kerslake A, Black J. Right to legal capacity in therapeutic jurisprudence: insights from critical disability theory and the convention on the rights of persons with disabilities. Int J Law Psychiatry. 2020;68:101535.

37. Potthoff S, Finke M, Scholten M, Gieselmann A, Vollmann J, Gather J. Opportunities and risks of self-binding directives: a qualitative study involving stakeholders and researchers in Germany. Front Psychiatry. 2022;13.
38. Eikelmann B. Sozialpsychiatrisches Basiswissen: Grundlagen und Praxis. Stuttgart: Enke; 1997.
39. Bolton D, Gillett G. The biopsychosocial model of health and disease: new philosophical and scientific developments. Cham: Palgrave; 2019.
40. Richter D. Chronic mental illness and the limits of the biopsychosocial model. Med Health Care Philos. 1999;2(1):21–30.
41. Read J, Bentall RP, Fosse R. Time to abandon the bio-bio-bio model of psychosis: exploring the epigenetic and psychological mechanisms by which adverse life events lead to psychotic symptoms. Epidemiol Psychiatr Sci. 2009;18(4):299–310.
42. Richter D, Dixon J. Models of mental health problems: a quasi-systematic review of theoretical approaches. J Ment Health. 2023;32(2):396–406.
43. Bech P, Olsen LR, Kjoller M, Rasmussen NK. Measuring well-being rather than the absence of distress symptoms: a comparison of the SF-36 mental health subscale and the WHO-five well-being scale. Int J Methods Psychiatr Res. 2003;12(2):85–91.
44. Leamy M, Bird V, Le Boutillier C, Williams J, Slade M. Conceptual framework for personal recovery in mental health: systematic review and narrative synthesis. Br J Psychiatry. 2011;199(6):445–52.
45. Annesley PT. Psychiatric illness in adolescence: presentation and prognosis. J Ment Sci. 1961;107(447):268–78.
46. Hirjak D, Leweke FM, Deuschle M, Staudter C, Borgwedel D, Coenen-Daniel M, et al. Das ZI-Track-Konzept in der modernen Psychiatrie: Eine syndromspezifische sektorenübergreifende Behandlung. Fortschritte der Neurologie und Psychiatrie. 2019;88(01):24–32.
47. Perkins A, Ridler J, Browes D, Peryer G, Notley C, Hackmann C. Experiencing mental health diagnosis: a systematic review of service user, clinician, and carer perspectives across clinical settings. Lancet Psychiatry. 2018;5(9):747–64.
48. Porter R. Madness: a brief history. Oxford: Oxford UP; 2013.
49. Schlichthorst M, Ozols I, Reifels L, Morgan A. Lived experience peer support programs for suicide prevention: a systematic scoping review. Int J Ment Heal Syst. 2020;14(1):65.
50. Burr C, Schnackenberg JK, Weidner F. Talk-based approaches to support people who are distressed by their experience of hearing voices: a scoping review. Front Psychiatry. 2022;13.
51. Torkildsen Ø. Lessons to be learnt from the history of lobotomy. Tidsskriftet den Norge Legeforening. 2022;142(18).
52. Scull A. Desperate remedies: psychiatry's turbulent quest to cure mental illness. Cambridge, MA: Harvard University Press; 2022.
53. Spiess M, Hotzy F, Ruffin R, Theodoridou A, Jäger M, Vogel U. Evaluation der Bestimmungen zur fürsorgerischen Unterbringung (FU; Art. 426 ff. ZGB). Bern: Bundesamt für Justiz; 2022.
54. Schlimme JE, Scholz T, Seroka R. Medikamentenreduktion und Genesung von Psychosen. Köln: Psychiatrie Verlag; 2018.
55. Rose D, MacDonald D, Wilson A, Crawford M, Barnes M, Omeni E. Service user led organisations in mental health today. J Ment Health. 2016;25(3):254–9.
56. Blenkiron P, Hammill CA. What determines patients' satisfaction with their mental health care and quality of life? Postgrad Med J. 2003;79(932):337–40.
57. Herek GM. Sexual orientation differences as deficits: science and stigma in the history of American psychology. Perspect Psychol Sci. 2010;5(6):693–9.
58. Priebe S, Omer S, Giacco D, Slade M. Resource-oriented therapeutic models in psychiatry: conceptual review. Br J Psychiatry. 2014;204(4):256–61.
59. Castel R. From dangerousness to risk. In: Scambler G, editor. Medical sociology: major themes in health and social welfare. IV: Health care and social change. London: Routledge; 2005. p. 235–50.

60. Robertson JP, Collinson C. Positive risk taking: whose risk is it? An exploration in community outreach teams in adult mental health and learning disability services. Health Risk Soc. 2011;13(2):147–64.
61. Burr C, Richter D. Zwischen Offenheit und Ablehnung - Die Einstellung von Psychiatriepflegenden gegenüber dem Risikoverhalten ihrer Patienten: eine qualitative Studie. Psychiatr Prax. 2017;44(6):348–55.
62. Puschner B, Becker T, Mayer B, Jordan H, Maj M, Fiorillo A, et al. Clinical decision making and outcome in the routine care of people with severe mental illness across Europe (CEDAR). Epidemiol Psychiatr Sci. 2016;25(1):69–79.
63. Gurtner C, Lohrmann C, Schols JMGA, Hahn S. Shared decision making in the psychiatric inpatient setting: an ethnographic study about interprofessional psychiatric consultations. Int J Environ Res Public Health. 2022;19(6):3644.
64. Gooding P. A new era for mental health law and policy: supported decision-making and the UN convention on the rights of persons with disabilities. Cambridge: Cambridge UP; 2017.
65. Forster R. Psychiatriereformen zwischen Medikalisierung und Gemeindeorientierung - Eine kritische Bilanz. Opladen: Westdeutscher Verlag; 1997.
66. Boardman J, Killaspy H, Mezey G. Social inclusion and mental health: understanding poverty, inequality and social exclusion. 2nd ed. Cambridge: Cambridge University Press; 2023.
67. Ankele M, Brinkschulte E, editors. Arbeitsrhythmus und Anstaltsalltag: Arbeit in der Psychiatrie vom frühen 19. Jahrhundert bis in die NS-Zeit. Stuttgart: Franz-Steiner-Verlag; 2015.
68. Ciompi L, Resultate und Prädiktoren der Rehabilitation. In: Hippius H, Lauter H, Ploog D, Bieber H, van Hout L, editors. Rehabilitation in der Psychiatrie. Heidelberg: Springer; 1988. p. 27–35.
69. Richter D, Hertig R, Hoffmann H. Psychiatrische Rehabilitation – von der Stufenleiter zur unterstützten Inklusion. Psychiatr Prax. 2016;43(8):444–9.
70. Beezhold J, Wise MJ, Eraslan D, Kastrup M. Informed consent in research settings. In: Fiorillo A, Volpe U, Bhugra D, editors. Psychiatry in practice: education, experience, and expertise. Oxford: Oxford University Press; 2016. p. 273–82.
71. Rose D. Mad Knowledges and user-led research. Cham: Palgrave Macmillan; 2022.
72. Gelfand T. Tuesdays at the SALPÊTRIÈRE. Bull Hist Med. 1989;63(1):132–6.
73. Happell B, Byrne L, McAllister M, Lampshire D, Roper C, Gaskin CJ, et al. Consumer involvement in the tertiary-level education of mental health professionals: a systematic review. Int J Ment Health Nurs. 2014;23(1):3–16.

Psychosocial Support Without Coercion: Consequences, Dilemmas and Possible Ways Out

8.1 Introduction

Although the current debate about the abolition of coercion through the UN Convention on the Rights of Persons with Disabilities continues to make waves, the demand is by no means new, even in professional circles. As early as 1999, the US Association of State Mental Health Programme Managers published a position paper that, while justifying the use of restraint in certain circumstances, formulated the goal of "… preventing, reducing and ultimately eliminating the use of seclusion and restraint…" [1]. This demand was met by many professional associations in the following years [2]. Interestingly, these demands were virtually uncontroversial at the time. This was possibly because the main focus was on reduction and not elimination.

The dispute began with the demand for the abolition of coercion. The possible abandonment of coercion in what we usually refer to today as mental health care was already described in the second chapter, with quotations from psychiatric professionals as quasi "inhumane" and a "historical step backwards". According to the conventional psychiatric interpretation, coercion protects people with mental disorders primarily in the context of endangering others and themselves.

From an empirical perspective, this connection between coercion and danger to oneself and others is not as compelling as it appears to be at first glance. With the abolition of psychiatric hospitals in Italy, there is, to a certain extent, a natural experiment [3]. It is well-known that inpatient bed capacity has significantly decreased in Italy since the end of the 1970s. However, unlike in many countries, this has not led to an increase in compulsory admissions; in contrast, it has actually led to a significant decrease. The same applies to forensic hospitalisation. Furthermore, the national suicide rate has not increased. Although coercion is still possible in psychiatric settings, developments have shown that a changed support system that involves less coercion does not automatically create "communicating pipes" that shift restrictive practices.

© The Author(s), under exclusive license to Springer Nature Switzerland AG 2025
D. Richter, *Human Rights in Psychiatry*,
https://doi.org/10.1007/978-3-031-98635-2_8

Nevertheless, a corresponding implementation of the UN CRPD would have considerable consequences, as it aims to completely abolish coercion in psychiatry. The American psychiatrist Paul Appelbaum, one of the most vehement critics of the UN CRPD, describes it with reference to criminal proceedings, saying that this would lead to convictions and prison sentences for people who were previously not considered responsible for their actions [4]. Many of those affected who are treated against their will in forensic hospitals today would therefore end up in prison, often without psychosocial support, as we know from the conditions in these institutions.

Even if I basically disagree with Appelbaum's fundamental opposition to the UN CRPD, in my opinion, he rightly criticises the fact that the proponents of the Convention remain silent about this issue. It concerns not only external endangerment and criminal behaviour, which are rarely mentioned but also self-harming and suicidal behaviour [5]. In my opinion, the advocates of the Convention are not doing themselves or the cause any favours by doing this, because they are allowing psychiatric critics a considerable and not easily refutable argument. If serious crimes were committed by people with psychosocial problems who could have been treated against their will, the public and the media would probably show no sympathy for this. The same applies, for example, to a possible suicide of a young adult who was in contact with psychiatric services but could not be held there involuntarily for reasons of the UN CRPD.

In the discussion to date about the abolition of coercion in psychiatry, the proponents therefore failed to analyse the obvious consequences and problems that such a step would entail. What consequences would this have for forensic psychiatry? How do we deal with people who want to take their own lives? How do we deal with people who are suffering from dementia? It is not only at first glance that the call for the abolition of coercion poses considerable dilemmas. If the abolition of coercion has a chance, these dilemmas and the associated difficulties must be addressed and analysed. This will be done below, at least to some extent. The following aspects will be analysed in detail: (1) the possible consequences of a preference-based declaration of being ill/not ill, (2) the possible consequences of preference-based psychosocial support, (3) the dilemmas associated with the removal of coercion in cases of aggression to others, and (4) the dilemmas associated with the renunciation of coercion in connection with suicidal tendencies and self-harm.

8.2 Consequences of a Preference-Oriented Self-Declaration of Ill/Not Ill

As a reminder, the justification for preference-based self-declaration was based on the empirical finding that an exclusive external declaration and diagnosis of "mental disorder" is based on insufficiently valid and sometimes arbitrary criteria. Nevertheless, the concept of a "mental illness" is widespread in modern society and is accepted by many people. However, there are also people who do not recognise this concept in general or for themselves in certain situations. This led to the conclusion that people should be able to decide for themselves whether they categorise themselves as "mentally ill" or "not ill" and therefore whether to make use of support services.

A corresponding self-declaration leads to various problems given the current conditions in the healthcare system and in the judiciary. Let us stay with the healthcare system first. The current situation is that medical, therapeutic, psychological, (usually also) nursing and (possibly also) social work support services are linked to a medical diagnosis. Without a diagnosis, i.e. without the identification of an illness, no healthcare services are financially covered by social insurance or other agencies. This even applies in the rehabilitation system, for example, with the rehabilitation classification ICF (*International Classification of Functioning, Disability and Health*), which must be assessed in conjunction with the ICD disease classification and which presupposes a health problem as a disease or disorder. Without the identification of a corresponding health problem, the ICF may not actually be used [6].

If the external identification of a mental illness was to be cancelled, the person would still be left to make the diagnosis and support services still be used. In this case, an expansion of services in certain areas is certainly to be expected. There would be cases in which people would want to make use of support that is currently not possible without a diagnosis. Apart from the question of the extent to which such support services would be offered and financed at all, the question arises as to whether this could generally lead to an expansion of services and an associated increase in costs. In my opinion, this is not certain. It is highly likely that support services that currently require a visit to a medical specialist would be less utilised and, thus, be reduced in the future. The costs of medicalising certain social problems would also be reduced.

The consequences for the judicial system would be serious. In court proceedings, it would be up to the accused person to determine whether they had carried out a certain act as part of a "mental illness". Should they refuse to do so, they would be subjected to regular proceedings without any diminished capacity diagnosed by others coming into play. In contrast to many myths surrounding diminished capacity, this does not lead to shorter sentences or quicker release [7]. As these people are commonly detained in forensic hospitals, where the placements are usually not scheduled in advance, this often leads to significantly longer sentences. This is not the only reason why many of those affected do not agree with the finding of diminished culpability.

As already mentioned, a major dilemma arises from the often inadequate psychosocial support in prisons. Psychosocial problems do not necessarily have to have been present before the start of the sentence; imprisonment itself can also trigger them. Suicides are known to occur significantly more frequently in prison populations than in the general population [8]. These effects should be seen in particular against the background of the unattainable goal of prison sentences. These sentences have virtually no effect on crime, as older [9] and more recent [10] empirical studies have repeatedly found. Their sole purpose is to keep people away from other people for a certain period of time, but they do not serve their supposed purpose of deterring the punished people from committing further offences.

If the person declares themselves to be "mentally ill", has committed an offence within the framework of diminished culpability and is willing to undergo treatment, then they would, to a certain extent, be undergoing voluntary psychiatric forensic treatment, which could be combined with a sentence. Voluntary forensic treatment is already not uncommon in outpatient settings in Switzerland [11]. However, there would certainly also be a need for inpatient facilities in which voluntary forensic treatment would be possible. Difficulties can arise if the opinion of the person concerned changes; then, the question is, what applies now: ill or not ill? Advance directives, in which the person concerned makes decisions, could help out of the dilemma here.

8.3 Consequences of Preference-Based Psychosocial Support

Preference-based psychosocial support has a certain connection with the question of being ill or not ill, but this is not mandatory. People who declare themselves to be ill may also prefer non-evidence-based interventions. Other people might choose to forgo the medical system from the outset and favour coaching or peer support that is not conventionally covered by health insurance. In addition, various combinations of evidence-based and non-evidence-based programmes are conceivable.

Such development presumably would not have any drastic consequences for the mental state of the general population. The current conventional and evidence-based psychiatric interventions do not leave any traces in terms of "better" health at the population level, as has been empirically established on various occasions [12, 13]. Therefore, even a less evidence-based development should not influence this.

Consequences could possibly be found in the economy. In relevant health economic research, substitution effects are assumed, as has been found for homeopathic and phytotherapeutic products [14]. This means that if certain preference-based medicines are prescribed, this could have a negative effect on other medicines, and vice versa. The key question would then be who finances which services. Would health insurance companies have to agree to everything that their policyholders wanted to use, even if the policyholders did not categorise themselves as "ill"? Or would it be up to the social insurance funds to finance services that the health insurance funds did not want, as these would not be medical services in the strictest sense?

One way out could be a defined catalogue of services that are preferred by people with psychosocial problems. Such a procedure would not be without precedent. Insured persons can already be reimbursed by health insurers for services that are considered preference-based rather than evidence-based. In Switzerland, for example, these services are subject to "medical complementary medicine" [15]. This includes acupuncture, anthroposophic medicine and homeopathy. In Germany, for example, homeopathy is also reimbursable by individual health insurance funds. In the area of social welfare, such catalogues and measures are also not without precedent. As part of the so-called subject financing of services for people with disabilities, which is about to be introduced in the canton of Bern, those affected can choose both services in defined areas and service providers [16]. However, to counteract a possible increase in volume, people must undergo a needs assessment. A similar instrument exists with the personal budget in Germany [17].

8.4 Harm to Others in a Psychosocial Support Programme Without Coercion

What should happen to people with psychosocial problems who may harm other people or who have actually physically assaulted others? In contrast to self-harm, which is analysed further below, modern society has a system that can, in principle, address all people who are danger to others. Police and judicial institutions are designed to deal with such difficult people and situations. Many people in prison have already been diagnosed as "mentally ill". Psychosis, severe depression and, above all, drug and alcohol problems are widespread in these institutions [8].

Why shouldn't the police and judiciary also be able to deal with people who are today admitted to a psychiatric hospital against their will because they are in danger to others and may be treated there? In my opinion, there is no fundamental argument against this. In addition, when I say in principle, I mean that under the current conditions, people with psychosocial problems are not in good hands in prisons. There is a widespread lack of appropriate support facilities to which people who endanger or have harmed other people are also entitled. This is one of the fundamental dilemmas that needs to be resolved if non-coercive psychosocial support is to be implemented in psychiatric settings.

I am sceptical as to whether this dilemma can be solved within the framework of current institutions for prisoners. We probably need a significantly different system for dealing with punishment in general. I have already mentioned that penalties do not have a major impact on criminal offences but can merely keep people with certain risks away for a certain period of time. Taking this further, a possible way out could be a "quarantine model". Philosophers Gregg Caruso [18] and Derk Pereboom [19] have developed this model in recent years as an alternative to the approach of morally justified punishments, as it is repeatedly advocated, especially in the United States.

The background to the quarantine model is the discussion about free will. Caruso and Pereboom fundamentally question the existence of free will. In contrast, they advocate the approach of "neuroexistentialism" [20]. According to this approach, all actions, decisions and experiences are biologically determined; a soul, a spirit or a corresponding consciousness as a non-physical something does not exist. "The universe is causally closed, and the mind is the brain" ([20]: 8). On the basis of this premise, neuroexistentialism concludes that people bear no moral responsibility for their actions and therefore cannot be punished for their crimes. However, people and societies are allowed to defend themselves against people who pose danger or risk. The quarantine model is then justified by analogy with the fight against epidemics. According to further arguments, it is permissible to keep people away from other people if they pose a danger, even if they are not responsible for this. We have often experienced this kind of approach with compulsory quarantine during the COVID-19 pandemic. People had to stay indoors after a proven infection to prevent them from passing on the infection.

In my opinion, the quarantine model can generally be applied to people who pose a danger to other people. It is also permissible to keep people with psychosocial problems away from other people if they are in danger to other people, for example, in the event of recurrence and according to relevant prognostic procedures. Moreover, the quarantine model is compatible because the placement must be as least restrictive as possible on the one hand and rehabilitative on the other hand. Caruso calls for rehabilitation to be organised according to the human rights capabilities approach of Martha Nussbaum and Amartya Sen [21]. Capabilities are opportunities for empowerment and realisation, for example, in terms of physical health, social relationships and control over one's own environment. These opportunities for empowerment and realisation are also required in psychiatric rehabilitation and are seen as the background for inclusion and recovery [22].

Furthermore, just as in psychiatric rehabilitation, Caruso calls for basic social conditions to be met, such as the right to housing, healthcare, sufficient income and more. In his view, these conditions are prerequisites for the prevention of criminal offences. In my opinion, they are also conditions for the prevention of some psychosocial problems, such as social exclusion and some mental health problems, in a narrow sense.

Whether and how a quarantine model can be implemented in practice is certainly doubtful under current conditions. However, from the perspective of psychosocial support without coercion outlined here, the model is attractive in various respects. First, there is no need to identify a "disorder" or "illness". Second, the focus is on rehabilitative goals. Third, involuntary therapies must be avoided at all costs. The punitive nature of the institution must be avoided as best as possible.

8.5 Self-Harm in a Psychosocial Support Programme Without Coercion

In contrast to harming others, there is no social institution or social system that could serve as an alternative to a psychiatric hospital in the case of life-threatening self-harm. Therefore, should there be no alternative to compulsory hospitalisation when dealing with suicidal behaviour? The World Health Organisation (WHO) and other UN organisations calling for the abolition of coercion are avoiding a clear answer to this question.

The initial situation regarding the prevention of suicide by coercion can be described as follows [23]: (1) coercive hospitalisations can save the lives of people who would certainly have committed suicide without intervention, (2) false-positive decisions for coercive interventions are unavoidable, as the prediction of suicide is very rarely reliably successful; many people are coercively hospitalised without actually having committed or attempting suicide, (3) the coercive nature of current psychiatric care alone will likely cause people to refrain from seeking support and

8.5 Self-Harm in a Psychosocial Support Programme Without Coercion

possibly commit suicide, and (4) a solution to coercion due to suicidal behaviour that is compatible with the UN CRPD is not apparent. Another complicating factor is that drug treatments [24] and psychosocial interventions also have no clear effects on the prevention of suicidal or self-harming behaviour [25]. The same applies to psychotherapeutic procedures [26] or brief contact interventions after discharge from inpatient treatment [27]. It is currently completely unclear how suicidal or self-harming behaviour can be effectively prevented [28].

These difficulties are also shared from the perspective of affected persons who have experienced suicidal behaviour. However, they make it clear that in conventional psychiatric care, there are virtually no opportunities to report their suicidal ideas or behaviour in a setting that is not associated with restrictive practices [29]. As already mentioned in the introduction, this situation is experienced as an epistemic injustice, and the associated *suicidism* is seen as pejorative discrimination and stigmatisation [30]. In this context, however, we are talking not only about epistemic injustice but also about epistemic violence inflicted on people who want to take their own lives [31].

It is therefore obvious to demand a right to self-chosen death that is not prevented or enabled by medical or disability-related criteria. Any application of medical or other criteria to medically assisted death is criticised in a new article by Alexandre Baril as *sanist* and *ableist* [32]. Baril consistently rejects a medically regulated practice of assisted suicide and instead calls for universal access to assisted suicide options.

Possible ways out of the current practice of attempting to prevent suicide can be derived from these points of view. First, there would need to be an expansion of options for assisted suicide, which would also be accessible to people with psychosocial problems. I myself have proposed making this possible for people who are not in an acute mental health crisis and have a well-considered wish to die [33]. I am convinced that it would be a fundamental task for professionals in the psychosocial support system to accompany people on this path.

Second, there needs to be a support system for people who are suicidal that does not include coercive measures. One approach in this regard is the "Wegloophuis" ("Runaway house") movement developed in the Netherlands in the 1970s [34]. These were facilities run and managed by people with lived experience in psychiatry. In Australia, various types of refuge centres have recently emerged, some of which are also integrated into regular funding. One option is the so-called "sub-acute recovery and prevention" approach. Its function is both to prevent acute psychiatric treatment and to provide a place that facilitates the transition into the community after acute psychiatric care is provided. A recent study of these facilities revealed that most affected individuals have improved in terms of recovery and that peer counselling in particular is considered very valuable [35].

Another option is a peer-led centre that is responsible for people experiencing suicidal crises. Those affected can stay in this "respite" centre for up to 4 days free of charge and are supported by peers as well as psychological specialists. Reviews have compared such crisis centres with conventional acute psychiatric settings in terms of various indicators and suggest that the crisis centres are rated significantly better by affected users [36]. However, it cannot be guaranteed on the basis of these studies that the characteristics of the people accompanied were identical.

To my knowledge, whether and to what extent non-psychiatric contact centres for people with suicidal thoughts could prevent such acts has not yet been thoroughly investigated. This would certainly be a worthwhile endeavour. In addition, the relationship between the psychosocial support system and suicidality should be discussed. In my opinion, prevention is not always the top priority. We must accept that people with and without psychosocial problems can see suicide as a legitimate way out of life.

8.6 Dementia and Psychosocial Support Without Coercion

A particular psychosocial problem that can be associated with both self-endangerment and endangerment of others is dementia, which is known to become more likely with increasing age. This problem is usually solved by determining the person's capacity, and in the event of a negative assessment, it is therefore legal and justified according to conventional ethics to carry out measures against the person's will.

Strictly applying the conditions of the UN CRPD is not permissible in principle. The person concerned retains their legal capacity even if they are presumed to be incapable of judgement from an external perspective and may refuse such measures.

One way out of this problem is advance directives. Such documents, which contain the will of the person, are already common in the care of people with dementia, for example, in the question of how to address life-prolonging measures [37]. The handling of coercion in certain situations could also be regulated in advance directives; these regulations could, for example, contain Ulysses clauses that make it possible to act against the will expressed in crisis situations. An advance directive of this kind can either be developed together with the person concerned in the event of the onset of dementia or, as in the case of organ donation in many countries, may even be used across the entire population.

In the case of indicated advance directives, it is necessary under certain circumstances to support them with professionals who have received training in the clinical picture, possible cognitive limitations and appropriate communication skills [38]. However, according to the relevant research, a one-off order is not enough. In a crisis situation, the "now-self" may no longer agree with the decisions of the "then-self" [39]. In this respect, the dispositions should be regularly evaluated with the person concerned and possibly revised. Research is currently being carried out into interaction procedures that go beyond the spoken word to give people with advanced dementia the opportunity to articulate their will [40].

8.7 Conclusions: Towards Psychosocial Support Without Coercion

The situations and dilemmas just described do not make us confident that psychosocial support without coercion could become a reality in the foreseeable future. From a sociological perspective, psychiatry without coercion has considerable consequences for various social systems and institutions. It would require not only a different understanding of "mental illness" but also a fundamentally different psychiatry. Such a fundamentally different psychiatry has recently been outlined by Diana Rose and her husband, sociologist Nicholas Rose. As a person with psychosocial problems herself, Diana Rose has analysed various reform proposals and made them herself. In the end, she and her husband arrive at the following characterisation of a "different psychiatry":

> More fundamentally it would invert the gaze through which distress was to be understood; it would require that all those professionals tried, in whatever way they could, to take the patient's point of view, to try to imagine the world as it is experienced by the patient. A move to epistemic justice demands that the voice of the patient and the experienced reality of the patient, is central to any system of supports and the holistic knowledge of actual lives that this would bring would render the idea of distinct 'components' redundant. Another psychiatry would be one that turns 'patient involvement in research' to 'researcher involvement in patient-led systems. ([41]: 7)

And that would not be enough. We would also need a changed legal and penal system and a drastically changed social law that no longer relies on a diagnosis to fund services. The medicalisation of the legal system is, in fact, one of the major obstacles on the way to abolishing coercion in psychiatry. Another obstacle is the public's positive attitude towards the medicalisation of problems. Linked to this is the widespread belief in the existence and validity of mental illness and psychiatric diagnoses. None of these can be changed quickly.

Until then, however, numerous initiatives could already be launched under the current legal and social conditions. These options range from open ward doors to home treatment, Open Dialogue and supported housing, runaway houses and peer respites, support for suicidal behaviour without coercion in the background, de-escalation and aggression management for all employees and advance directives. These are all topics that can already be realised today without immediately calling for a different psychiatry. The first step would be to consistently implement the ethical demands for the least possible restrictions and coercion as a last resort.

The abolition of coercion in mental health settings will not happen from one day to the next. However, the path should be inevitable.

References

1. NASMHPD. Position statement on seclusion and restraint: National Association of State Mental Health Program Directors 1999. Available from: https://www.nasmhpd.org/content/position-statement-seclusion-and-restraint.

2. Zaami S, Rinaldi R, Bersani G, Marinelli E. Restraints and seclusion in psychiatry: striking a balance between protection and coercion – critical overview of international regulations and rulings. Riv Psichiatr. 2020;55(1):16–23.
3. Barbui C, Papola D, Saraceno B. Forty years without mental hospitals in Italy. Int J Ment Heal Syst. 2018;12(1):43.
4. Appelbaum PS. Protecting the rights of persons with disabilities: an international convention and its problems. Psychiatr Serv. 2016;67(4):366–8.
5. Duffy RM, Kelly BD. Rights, laws and tensions: a comparative analysis of the convention on the rights of persons with disabilities and the WHO resource book on mental health, human rights and legislation. Int J Law Psychiatry. 2017;54:26–35.
6. Kostanjsek N, Rubinelli S, Escorpizo R, Cieza A, Kennedy C, Selb M, et al. Assessing the impact of health conditions using the ICF. Disabil Rehabil. 2011;33(15–16):1475–82.
7. Perlin ML. The insanity defense: nine myths that will not go away. In: White MD, editor. The insanity defense: multidisciplinary views on its history, trends, and controversies. Santa Barbara: Praeger/ABC-CLIO; 2016. p. 3–22.
8. Fazel S, Hayes AJ, Bartellas K, Clerici M, Trestman R. Mental health of prisoners: prevalence, adverse outcomes, and interventions. Lancet Psychiatry. 2016;3(9):871–81.
9. Gendreau P, Cullen FT, Goggin C. The effects of prison sentences on recidivism. Ottawa: Solicitor General Canada; 1999.
10. Beckett K, Goldberg A. The effects of imprisonment in a time of mass incarceration. Crime Justice. 2022;51:349.
11. Krammer S, Gamma A, Znoj H, Klecha D, Signorini P, Liebrenz M. Effectiveness of forensic outpatients' psychiatric treatment and recidivism rates: a comparison study. Forensic Sci Int Mind Law. 2020;1:100032.
12. Richter D, Wall A, Bruen A, Whittington R. Is the global prevalence rate of adult mental illness increasing? Systematic review and meta-analysis. Acta Psychiatr Scand. 2019;140(5):393–407.
13. Ormel J, Hollon SD, Kessler RC, Cuijpers P, Monroe SM. More treatment but no less depression: the treatment-prevalence paradox. Clin Psychol Rev. 2022;91:102111.
14. Bauer C, Giulini-Limbach C, May U, Schneider-Ziebe A, Abels C, Walendzik A, et al. Versorgungspolitische und gesundheitsökonomische Aspekte zum Regulierungsstatus homöopathischer Arzneimittel. IBES Diskussionsbeitrag; 2021.
15. Etter G. Komplementärmedizin–10 Jahre nach der Abstimmung. Bulletin des médecins suisses. 2019;100(2324):795.
16. BZ. Mehr Selbstbestimmung für Menschen mit Behinderung. Berner Zeitung 2022 07-12-2022.
17. Sobota R. Leitfaden Persönliches Budget. Köln: Psychiatrie Verlag/BALANCE; 2012.
18. Caruso GD. Rejecting retributivism: free will, punishment, and criminal justice. Cambridge: Cambridge UP; 2021.
19. Pereboom D. Free will skepticism and prevention of crime. In: Pereboom D, Shaw E, Caruso GD, editors. Free will skepticism in law and society: challenging retributive justice. Cambridge: Cambridge University Press; 2019. p. 99–115.
20. Caruso G, Flanagan O, editors. Neuroexistentialism: meaning, morals, and purpose in the age of neuroscience. Oxford: Oxford University Press; 2017.
21. Nussbaum M. Human rights and human capabilities. Harvard Human Rights J. 2007;20:21–4.
22. Richter D. Inklusion, Exklusion und Integration: Schlüsselkonzepte für die psychiatrische (Arbeits-) Rehabilitation. In: Kawohl W, Rössler W, editors. Arbeit und Psyche: Grundlagen, Therapie, Rehabilitation, Prävention - Ein Handbuch. Stuttgart: Kohlhammer; 2018. p. 94–106.
23. Wang DWL, Colucci E. Should compulsory admission to hospital be part of suicide prevention strategies? BJPsych Bull. 2017;41(3):169–71.
24. Huang X, Harris LM, Funsch KM, Fox KR, Ribeiro JD. Efficacy of psychotropic medications on suicide and self-injury: a meta-analysis of randomized controlled trials. Transl Psychiatry. 2022;12(1):400.
25. Itzhaky L, Davaasambuu S, Ellis SP, Cisneros-Trujillo S, Hannett K, Scolaro K, et al. Twenty-six years of psychosocial interventions to reduce suicide risk in adolescents: systematic review and meta-analysis. J Affect Disord. 2022;300:511–31.

26. Teismann T, Gysin-Maillart A. Psychotherapie nach einem Suizidversuch—Evidenzlage und Bewertung. Bundesgesundheitsbl Gesundheitsforsch Gesundheitsschutz. 2022;65(1):40–6.
27. Tay JL, Li Z. Brief contact interventions to reduce suicide among discharged patients with mental health disorders—a meta-analysis of RCTs. Suicide Life Threat Behav. 2022;52(6):1074–95.
28. Fox KR, Huang X, Guzmán EM, Funsch KM, Cha CB, Ribeiro JD, et al. Interventions for suicide and self-injury: a meta-analysis of randomized controlled trials across nearly 50 years of research. Psychol Bull. 2020;146(12):1117–45.
29. Webb D. Re-conceptualizing suicidality: towards collective intersubjective responses. In: Beresford P, Russo J, editors. The Routledge international handbook of mad studies. Londeon: Routledge; 2021. p. 243–52.
30. Baril A. Suicidism: a new theoretical framework to conceptualize suicide from an anti-oppressive perspective. Disabil Stud Q. 2020;40(3).
31. Wedlake G. Complicating theory through practice: affirming the right to die for suicidal people. Can J Disabil Stud. 2020;9(4):89–110.
32. Baril A. Theorizing the intersections of ableism, sanism, ageism and suicidism in suicide and physician-assisted death debates. The disability bioethics reader. London: Routledge; 2022. p. 221–31.
33. Richter D. Unerträgliches Leiden und autonome Entscheidung: Warum Menschen mit psychischen Erkrankungen das Recht auf Sterbehilfe nicht verwehrt werden darf. In: Böhning A, editor. Assistierter Suizid für psychisch Erkrankte: Herausforderung für Psychiatrie und Psychotherapie. Bern: Hogrefe; 2021. p. 37–61.
34. Verhey TC. Het Wegloophuis Huisarts en Wetenschap. 1987;30:70–1.
35. Waks S, Morrisroe E, Reece J, Fossey E, Brophy L, Fletcher J. Consumers lived experiences and satisfaction with sub-acute mental health residential services. Soc Psychiatry Psychiatr Epidemiol. 2024;59(10):1849–59.
36. Smithson JS. Efficacy of mental health crisis houses compared with acute mental health wards: a literature review. Ment Health Pract. 2019;27(4).
37. Harrison Dening K, Sampson EL, De Vries K. Advance care planning in dementia: recommendations for healthcare professionals. Palliat Care Res Treat. 2019;12:1178224219826579.
38. Dixon J, Laing J, Valentine C. A human rights approach to advocacy for people with dementia: a review of current provision in England and Wales. Dementia. 2020;19(2):221–36.
39. Opgenhaffen T, Put J, Lepeleire JD, Keady J, Swinnen A. Care planning and the lived experience of dementia: establishing real will and preferences beyond mental capacity. In: Schokkaert E, Vandenbulcke M, Dröes R-M, editors. Dementia and society. Cambridge: Cambridge University Press; 2022. p. 211–32.
40. Keady JD, Campbell S, Clark A, Dowlen R, Elvish R, Jones L, et al. Re-thinking and re-positioning 'being in the moment' within a continuum of moments: introducing a new conceptual framework for dementia studies. Ageing Soc. 2022;42(3):681–702.
41. Rose D, Rose N. Is 'another' psychiatry possible? Psychol Med. 2023;53(1):46–54.

Epilogue: On the Way to a Post-liberal Psychiatry? 9

9.1 Text

As much as I am convinced that psychiatry with coercive measures cannot be justified and that psychiatry without coercion must ultimately come, I realise in the spring of 2025, when this manuscript is completed, that a liberal psychiatry without restrictions will have a difficult time in the foreseeable future. Human rights are currently hardly being promoted, especially in psychiatry, and in many cases, we are even seeing a roll-back towards a post-liberal psychiatry.

In many countries, there has been a significant increase in coercive psychiatric measures, as I mentioned in the introductory chapter. Despite all these assurances, human rights in psychiatry are less protected in everyday clinical practice today than they were a few years ago. At the same time, we are witnessing a significant expansion of forensic institutions in many countries [1]. There are also calls to re-establish psychiatric asylum in a modernised form [2].

In Europe, we are experiencing a debate about how to deal with offenders who appear to have psychosocial problems. In connection with attacks by individuals on the civilian population, the call for surveillance of people with psychoses is growing louder, particularly among conservative politicians.

In the United States, a discussion about the treatment of homeless people who I find very worrying has recently developed. In administrations governed by Democrats such as California and New York City, of all places, homelessness is seen as an indication for compulsory psychiatric hospitalisation. As much as I recognise the problem of homelessness and the associated psychosocial problems on the American West Coast and in many larger cities, the wrong priorities are clearly being set here. It is, as observers have already noted, a medicalisation of social problems [3]. An inadequate housing policy and an insufficiently functioning welfare state cannot be compensated for by coercive psychiatric measures.

However, these measures are certainly appreciated by the public. In California, the population voted on measures to combat homelessness in a referendum. The budget for the expansion of psychiatric treatment centres far exceeded the budget for housing. The proposal initiated by the state of California was—narrowly—accepted.

This indicates that measures against a person's will are also accepted in more liberal circles. The question is, how did this come about? In my opinion, three main aspects are important here. First, "mental illnesses" are now predominantly viewed in the same way as physical illnesses. This also means that affected people should be treated accordingly. In addition, if this means treating those affected against their will, many in the general population apparently have no problem with this. The destigmatisation of mental health problems has negative consequences insofar as psychiatric coercion is generally regarded as standard treatment.

Second, and more importantly, even the liberal-minded population is increasingly less willing to accept disturbing behaviour by people with psychosocial problems. We in the social psychiatry community have seemingly overestimated society's tolerance. Moreover, a tolerant society, in psychiatric terms, needs the assurance that sufficient financial resources and staff are available to address the sometimes unpleasant and disturbing side effects of psychosocial problems. As long as we cannot ensure that these resources are sufficiently available, we cannot hope for continued tolerance towards people with psychosocial problems.

Finally, and third, we have obviously underestimated the resistance of conventional professional psychiatric associations and institutions. Despite all lip service, a psychiatric system that does not want to do without coercion is actually being developed further. To a certain extent, however, this is also due to the social psychiatry community. We have obviously not been sufficiently successful in developing alternatives for dealing with "difficult" situations in connection with psychosocial problems and establishing these alternatives in practice.

The ethical and empirical arguments that I have put forward here do not support this path. One can only hope that the phase of post-liberal psychiatry remains a brief intermezzo.

References

1. Chow WS, Priebe S. How has the extent of institutional mental healthcare changed in Western Europe? Analysis of data since 1990. BMJ Open. 2016;6(4):e010188.
2. Sisti DA, Segal AG, Emanuel EJ. Improving long-term psychiatric care: bring back the asylum. JAMA. 2015;313(3):243–4.
3. Zimmerman A. Homelessness and mental illness: medicalizing a housing crisis. J Human Rights Social Work. 2024;9(1):117–28.

MIX
Papier aus verantwortungsvollen Quellen
Paper from responsible sources
FSC® C105338

If you have any concerns about our products,
you can contact us on
ProductSafety@springernature.com

In case Publisher is established outside the EU,
the EU authorized representative is:
**Springer Nature Customer Service Center GmbH
Europaplatz 3, 69115 Heidelberg, Germany**

Printed by Libri Plureos GmbH
in Hamburg, Germany